David D Plain

Ways of Our Grandfathers

Our Traditions and Culture

To: My wife Gisele who is so patient and forgiving with all my quirks and little idiosyncrasies

Cover: "Indian Encampment on Lake Huron" by Paul Kane ca. 1848-52. Original painting at the Art Gallery of Ontario, Toronto, Canada. Photo image courtesy of Wikimedia Commons.

Order this book online at www.trafford.com/07-0677
or email orders@trafford.com

Most Trafford titles are also available at major online book retailers.

Note for Librarians: A cataloguing record for this book is available from Library and Archives Canada at www.collectionscanada.ca/amicus/index-e.html

ISBN: 978-1-4251-2276-8

We at Trafford believe that it is the responsibility of us all, as both individuals and corporations, to make choices that are environmentally and socially sound. You, in turn, are supporting this responsible conduct each time you purchase a Trafford book, or make use of our publishing services. To find out how you are helping, please visit www.trafford.com/responsiblepublishing.html

Our mission is to efficiently provide the world's finest, most comprehensive book publishing service, enabling every author to experience success. To find out how to publish your book, your way, and have it available worldwide, visit us online at www.trafford.com/10510

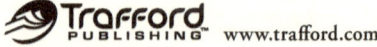 www.trafford.com

North America & international
toll-free: 1 888 232 4444 (USA & Canada)
phone: 250 383 6864 ♦ fax: 250 383 6804 ♦ email: info@trafford.com

The United Kingdom & Europe
phone: +44 (0)1865 722 113 ♦ local rate: 0845 230 9601
facsimile: +44 (0)1865 722 868 ♦ email: info.uk@trafford.com

10 9 8 7 6 5 4 3 2 1

Contents

4

Religious Life

Appendices

Illustrations (following 42)

Preface

I wrote *Ways of Our Grandfathers* to complement my book The Plains of Aamjiwnaang and I have made every effort to capture Ahnishenahbek culture from the pre and early contact periods. My family claims a long line of chiefs and so we are intrinsically leaders shaping Ahnishenahbek culture and determining our history.

We used the word Ahnishenahbek to describe ourselves as a people. Other names we have been known by include Ojibwa and Chippewa. Today Ahnishenahbek is used in several different ways, to describe our nation or to describe any member of the Three Fires Confederacy and sometimes in an even wider sense to describe any aboriginal people. In this publication I will use it to only describe our Nation or one of our member bands. Concerning grammar, spelling and capitalization I have not endeavoured to correct any errors made in any quotations I have used but left them intact.

Nicholas Plain Jr., my father, was an elected chief of Aamjiwnaang. His father, Ozahshkedawa (Out On the Plain), was the last traditional chief before the electoral system was imposed upon us under an amendment to the Indian Act in 1884. His father, Misquahwegezhigk (Red Sky) was a chief from

Aamjiwnaang. His father, Animikeence (Little Thunder) was both a war chief and a civil chief, as was his father, Kioscance (Young Gull). I will concentrate on the culture of Kioscance's time, which spanned pre and early contact periods.

Ways of the Grandfathers will probe the many different facets of the traditional lifestyle of the Ahnishenahbek. This book explores characteristics of political structure, worldview, dress and lifestyle including some food recipes, games and stories as well as providing an explanation of totems and wampum. It also describes economic life including trade and hunting, fishing and sugar camps. The final chapter deals with language and religion including death customs as well as traditional medicines.

I have spent many hours studying first hand accounts and source documents as well as listening to oral history as told by elders such as my father and my uncle Levi Plain. I was fortunate as a boy to be able to sit at the feet of these two grand old men and listen as they visited on our front porch on Exmouth Street. Their knowledge of our culture as told through traditional oral stories was vast. They personally practiced the old ways and their memories stretched back into the nineteenth century. They also related accounts of the way we lived, gathered from their mentors whose memories dated back to the beginnings of the reserve era.

I am also indebted to earlier cultural anthropologists who provided source documents such as the Jesuit Relations and Allied Documents, which contain excellent eyewitness accounts. Also much can be gleaned from the Wisconsin Historical Society and the Michigan Historical Society collections. The World Wide Web has opened up a whole new avenue for research, which I also found invaluable. I would especially like to mention the University of Toronto's web site "Early Canadiana", the University of Central Michigan's Clark

Historical Library site and the University of Indiana's "Miami Indians Ethnohistory Archives." I sincerely hope this book finds favour in your sight and that it will serve as a source of knowledge of Ahnishenahbek culture.

David D. Plain

Aamjiwnaang First Nation Territory

January 2007.

1

Characteristics

Description

From first contact with the Europeans the Ahnishenahbek were looked upon as "hospitable, proud, redoubtable to their enemies" and "very industrious ... the tribe had many brave warriors. These were feared and respected by all the other tribes around the Great Lakes. Warriors of this tribe were among the first in historic times to defeat the Iroquois."[1] The first to make contact with the Ahnishenahbek was Samuel de Champlain. He called us Cheveux-Relevés or the 'high hairs'. After "having visiting seven or eight of their villages [Petun], the explorers pushed forward still further west, when they came to the settlement of an interesting tribe, which they named 'Cheveux-Relevés' or the 'lofty haired', an appellation suggested by the mode of dressing their hair."[2] They are described as follows:

---

[1] Vernon W. Kinietz, *The Indians of the Western Great Lakes 1615-1760* (Ann Arbor: University of Michigan Press, 1940; Ann Arbor Paperback, 1991), 320-21.

[2] Samuel de Champlain, *Voyages of Samuel de Champlain 1537-1635*,

These are savages that wear nothing about the loins, and go stark naked, except in the winter, when they clothe themselves in robes of skins, which they leave off when they quit their houses for the fields. They are great hunters, fishermen, and travellers, till the soil, and plant Indian corn. They dry bluets [blueberries] and raspberries, in which they carry on an extensive traffic with other tribes, taking in exchange skins, beads, nets, and other articles. Some of these people pierce their nose, and attach beads to it. They tattoo their bodies, applying black and other colours. They wear their hair very straight, and grease it, painting it red, as they do also the face.[3]

The political structure of the Ahnishenahbek Nation was extremely flat. Each band, indeed each village had total autonomy. Each village had a council, which was made up of elders. Village councils invited its members to sit according to ability and demonstrated wisdom. Thus each village was self-governing led by the community's collective wisdom. The council was the only governing body to have coercive power. The council invited chiefs to their positions. They were chosen according to their demonstrative potential and had only charismatic power. For example, it was the council that determined support for a war effort, not the War Chief. It was the War Chief's responsibility to raise the warriors and he did this by depending on his charismatic abilities to instil a desire to

---

Vol. 1, trans. Charles Pomeroy Otis Ph.D. (Boston: The Prince Society, 1880), 139 available from http://www.canadiana.org/ECO/ItemRecord/26911?id=608edce981ea4 d7a last accessed 20 July 2006.

[3] Ibid., 303.

follow him into war. Incidentally, wars were almost always localized skirmishes between an individual band and a linguistically different neighbour.

There were also Civil Chiefs, who were responsible for such decisions as trade negotiations and in conjunction with War Chiefs, peace negotiations. Civil Chiefs were always good orators and they were the ones chosen to speak for the council at meetings with other nations. They were usually men but sometimes women could serve. Occasionally a single person could be both a War and a Civil chief.

The Ahnishenahbek did belong to an alliance with the Otahwah and the Potawatomi called the Three Fires Confederacy. When this alliance met it was called a Grand-Council and members were chosen by their village council to represent each village. Any member could call a Grand-Council to discuss any situation that might affect any or all of the three member nations.

The Ahnishenahbek arrived at Aamjiwnaang shortly after the Iroquois War. During the Traditional Period ca 1700-1827 we lived the traditional semi-nomadic life. The main villages were located on the east side of the St. Clair River at present day Sarnia and at the mouth of the Black River now Port Huron, Michigan. Our ancestors would spend the summer and fall collectively hunting, fishing and gathering. During this time they would also make trips to Fort Pontchartrain [Detroit] to trade pelts for European goods. After the fall gatherings [Powwows], usually held at Bawitig, (where Lakes Superior, Michigan and Huron converge) most would disperse into our hunting territory in smaller groups to spend the winter hunting and trapping. In the months of February and March they would move to their sugar camps to make maple sugar products, which they used for cooking and for trade. They then moved to their fishing camps for the spring fish runs and after this they all returned to congregate at the main villages for the summer and fall.

It is said by some modern historians that the First Nations were great stewards of the land and were among the earth's first conservationists. These kinds of statements are the result of a lack of understanding of First Nation philosophy. We did not see ourselves as somehow separate from nature with a need to "look after it". This is a modern, western concept that flows out of their earlier Biblical based idea that they were to "have dominion and subdue" the earth and its resources. Instead we saw ourselves as being an integral part of nature. Indeed, we even saw ourselves as being the weakest part needing both the Creator's help through the mahnedoog and the help of the game itself. We believed that animals had the ability to choose whether to give their lives for the sustenance of the people, which they often did according to the wishes of the Creator. Hence, we followed the practice of giving a tobacco offering when game was taken or for the use of resources such as trees for shelter or utensils.

Our philosophy was Platonic in nature. We thought that the physical world we lived in was only an image of the real world. The link between the two lay in dreams. So this made dreams and their interpretations extremely important and we lived our daily lives accordingly.

Language[4]

There were three linguistic groups living in the Great Lakes Basin interacting with the Ahnishenahbek nation. They were

---

[4] Richard Rhodes. *Eastern Ojibwa-Chippewa-Ottawa Dictionary* (New York: Mouton de Gruyter, 1993) x, xi, xxiv, xxv.

Siouan, Iroquoian and Algonquian speaking peoples. Some examples of nations speaking a Sioux language were Dakota, Lakota, Nakota, and Otchente Chakowin. The Winnebago or Puants were also of the Siouan linguistic group as were the Assiniboin. The nations speaking Iroquoian were the Huron, the Tobacco Nation (Tionontati) the Neutral Nation, the Erie and the St. Lawrence Iroquois. Members of the Five Nation Confederacy also spoke Iroquoian languages. These were the Mohawk, Onondaga, Oneida, Cayuga and Seneca nations.

The largest linguistic group in the area was by far the Algonquian group. Speakers of this language stock included the Cree, Menominee, Sauk, Fox, Kickapoo, Miami, Illinois, Shawanee, and Delaware, as well as the members of the Three Fires Confederacy, the Ahnishenahbek (Chippewa), Otahwah and Potawatomi. By the time we moved into Aamjiwnaang the Erie, St. Lawrence, and Neutral Iroquois had disappeared and the remnants of the Huron and Tionontati had merged to become the Wyandotte. One can see by these lists the diversity of languages spoken in the Great Lakes area.

The Ahnishenahbek language was so close to the Otahwah language that the two had no trouble understanding one another. In fact Otahwah is really an Ahnishenahbek dialect that had deviated farthest, but still belongs to the Southern Ahnishenahbek group of dialects. "The Ottawa dialect is also known as Chippewa or Ojibwa in Michigan and the adjacent region of Southern Ontario. This comes from the fact that many speakers of Ottawa there are descendents of Chippewas who, during the 1800's, moved into areas where Ottawa was the dialect spoken. Sometimes Ottawa speakers will say that the language they speak is a mixture of Ottawa and Chippewa ... which reflects a linguistic reality arising from the historical fact."[5]

The southern group also includes Eastern Ahnishenahbek. Eastern Ahnishenahbek is the dialect spoken on the eastern shore of Georgian Bay east to the Algonquin dialect, which for example is spoken on the Golden Lake and Maniwaki reserves.

There are two other distinct groups of Ahnishenahbek dialects. There is a northern group comprising of Severn Ahnishenahbek in Northern Ontario (know locally as Cree) and the Algonquin group mentioned above, which is spoken in South-western Quebec. The dialect spoken by the Ahnishenahbek of Aamjiwnaang like other Ahnishenahbek dialects were no doubt impacted by the interjection of Potawatomi words brought by the Potawatomi who settled among us in the 1800's.

There are a large number of variations heard among Ahnishenahbek speakers. They range from differences in pronunciation to varying forms of the same words to entirely different words and even different constructions are found. Some variations are personal in nature and some are a result of different ethnic or geographic roots. For example, all Otahwah and Ahnishenahbek speakers pronounce b, d, g, etc. at the end of words as if they were p, t, k, and etc. respectively. So they pronounce naasaab (the same) as though it were naasaap, and kaad (leg) as kaat. Speakers of Eastern Ahnishenahbek never do this. Every community has variations within it, as do individual families. For example, some speakers pronounce the word meaning winter as poon, or boon or bboon.

A speaker's choice of some words can distinguish the dialect he or she is speaking very clearly. For example, Otahwah and Ahnishenahbek speakers call the sugar maple sinaamizh, but

[5] Rhodes, *Eastern Ojibwa*, x, xi.

Eastern Ahnishenahbek speakers call the sugar maple ninaatig. Sometimes the choice of word occurs with a dialect. For example, some Otahwah and Ahnishenahbek speakers will call a tool aabjichgan while others call it nokaazwin. Likewise most Eastern Ahnishenahbek speakers call a table wiisniwaagan but some call it doopwin.

There are many English words borrowed by the Ahnishenahbek speaker. Generally speaking the further north the community the less borrowing is seen. U.S. Otahwah or Ahnishenahbek speakers will call electricity 'power' while Ontario speakers borrow the word 'hydro'. Some borrowed words that contain r or l undergo an adjustment toward Ojibwa phonology. For example, Mary or Marie becomes Maanii and Charlie becomes Chaalii. This applies to the letter v as well. My name is David as is my son's. At Aamjiwnaang we are called Chi-Dabid (Big David) and Dabidiins (Little David) respectively. Time is told in English but the hour is expressed as 'clock' not 'o'clock'. . What time is it? Two o'clock is expressed Aanii-sh e-piichi-yaag? Two Clock in Ahnishenahbewissin.

Band Designations, Totems and Wampum

Each band had its own hunting territory and these territories were given their own appellations to identify them. Some examples of these were given in the above section on the Iroquois War. For example, we were called Bawitigwakinini and we were one of the better-known bands. This is only because of our location, which was around the Falls of St. Mary's at Sault Ste. Marie. Bawitig means falls or rapids and inini denotes man. The suffix wak makes it plural. This word translates as People of the Falls or more literally Men of the Falls. Oumisagai or Eagle People were located south of the Bawitigwakinini on the north shore of Georgian Bay. Amikouai were known as the

Beaver People, Amik meaning Beaver. They were located south of Oumisagai.[6] Ketchesebewininewug were the Great River Men because they lived on the Banks of the Mississippi River.[7] As can be seen by this abbreviated list some of these bands had some animal either mammal, fish, bird or reptile embedded in their names and some had some other feature. This is because the names give some clue as to the location of the band's hunting territory, whether they lived near great rapids or good beaver hunting territory. Although the French used these appellations freely they referred collectively to the different bands of Ahnishenahbek as Ojibwa.

Band appellations can be very confusing when trying to trace band movements. Our names could change or even disappear which often happened when we expanded or relocated. Or sometimes we took our names with us. Sometimes we changed our band's name to describe some feature of our new location. For example, when we as a part of Bawitigwakinini expanded to Southeast Michigan we split into two bands. One of the bands called themselves Mekadewagamitigwayawininiwak or Men at the end of the Black River. The other Band called themselves Wapisiwisibwininiwak or Men of Swan Creek. Yet the French still referred to us as Sauteurs. When the Amikouai expanded south of Georgian Bay the band that moved into Saugeen Territory became know as Saugeewinini meaning "I am of the People of the River

---

[6] For a complete list of locations of Ojibwa Bands see *The Jesuit Relations and Allied Documents*, Vol. 18, Reuben Gold Thwaites, ed., (Cleveland: Burrows Bros. Pub., 1898), 227-235.

[7] William W. Warren, *History of the Ojibway People* (St. Paul: Minnesota Historical Society Press, vol. 5, 1885; Borealis Books, 1984), 39. Warren provides a complete list of Ojibway Bands located in the United States.

Mouth".[8]

These band names were in full use during the seventeenth century but fell out of use by the European record keepers during the eighteenth century. When the British became the dominant European power after defeating the French at Quebec in 1760 they ceased using the old appellations (except for the Mississauga) referring to Ahnishenahbek as Chippewa. However, Ahnishenahbek Bands still use some descriptive appellation even today. For example, Aamjiwnaang njibaad meaning I am from a place of tumbling waters (Sarnia) or Bkejwanong njibaad meaning I am from a place where the waters divide (Walpole Island).

To add to the confusion we also used symbols to designate the armorial sign different warrior groups fought under. For example, in a 1736 "Census of the Indian Tribes"[9] an enumeration is given of the nations connected with Canada giving their location, number of warriors and armorial bearings. In this census Sauteurs were located at Keweenaw, Point Chagouamigon and the Falls of Saint Mary and have three war devices. They are the Crane, the Catfish and the Stag. The Crane and Catfish were the devices of the Keweenaw Sauteurs and the Crane and the Stag were the emblems of the Sauteurs at the falls. No device was given for Point Chagouamigon.

The Otahwah were located at Michilimackinac, Saginaw and Detroit and each location had for their devices the Bear and the Black Squirrel. The Potawatomi were located on a small island in Lake Michigan, on the Saint Joseph River and at Detroit.

---

[8] Basil Johnston, *Ojibway Heritage*, (McClelland and Stewart, Toronto: 1974), 59-60.

[9] 1736: *Census of the Indian Tribes, Wisconsin Historical Society,,* vol. 17, 245-252.

They had for their armorial bearings the Golden Carp, the Frog, the Crab and the Tortoise. The census located the Mississauga at the River Mississauga, on Manitoulin Island, Lake Ontario and at Lake Saint Clair. They all have for a war device a Crane. These armorial signs are not to be confused with family totems.

In Ahnishenahbek culture there are two essential questions when introductions are made between strangers. The premier question and the one always asked first is "Waenaesh k'dodaem" meaning what is your totem.[10] Totems were family marks. They were almost always a pictogram of an animal, either a mammal, bird, fish or reptile and denoted which family an individual belonged to. During the surrender treaty period chiefs and principal men of the different bands used totems as a sign of their speaking authority for their families. The chiefs would make their totem mark on the document and the government agent would write their personal names phonetically beside their marks. The second question was "Waenaesh keen?" meaning who are you? The answer provided would be one of band membership such as the examples above.

According to tradition in the beginning there were only five totems and they were a gift from the spirit beings. Warren relates the traditional story this way:

> When the earth was new, the An-ish-in-aub-ag lived, congregated on the shores of a great salt water. From the bosom of the great deep there suddenly appeared six beings in human form who entered their wigwams.
>
> One of these six strangers kept a covering over his eyes, and he dared not look on the An-ish-in-aub-ag, though he showed the greatest anxiety to do so. At

[10] Ibid.,59.

last he could no longer restrain his curiosity, and on one occasion he partially lifted his veil, and his eye fell on the form of a human being, who instantly fell dead as if struck by one of the thunderers. Though the intentions of this dread being were friendly to the An-ish-in-aub-ag, yet the glance of his eye was too strong, and inflicted certain death. His fellows, therefore, caused him to return into the bosom of the great water from which they had apparently emerged.

The others, who now numbered five, remained with the An-ish-in-aub-ag and became a blessing to them; from them originate the five great clans or Totems, which are known among the Ojibways by the general terms of A-Wause-e, Bus-in-aus-e, Ah-ah-wauk, Noka, and Monsone or Waub-ish-ash-e. These are cognomens which are used only in connection with the Totemic system.[11]

Some researchers confuse band designations with totems because often band designations have some animal or bird rooted in the band name. Sometimes clans are referred to but totems are strictly family marks. Some of the different families may be more closely related and Warren mentions this by calling them great families. He gives the example of some of the smaller fish totems being closely related or belonging to one of the largest families, the Awause family, who claim the Meshemunaigway (immense fish) as their totem.[12]

I personally do not like the word clan because it is a borrowed word and evokes a western mentality with the

---

[11] Warren, *History*, 44.

[12] Ibid.,46.

concept of a hierarchical societal structure where nations are made up tribes and clans, and families. European clans have a coat of arms and keep strict track of family branches. Clan members could be related either closely or distantly. Distant relatives could marry even though they were from the same clan.

Some have taken this model and tried to superimpose it on Ahnishenahbek society. But our society was very flatly organized. Families were the backbone of the nation with each family represented in many bands. This, along with a common language, is what held the Ahnishenahbek together. Individuals with the same totem, no matter how remote the bands were to each other and even if they did not know each other, were considered close relatives. No member of the same totem was a distant relation. We used close relative names such as sister for sister-in-law and brother for brother-in-law. We used totems in the marriage tradition to prevent intermarriage. It was a highly immoral act to marry one from the same totem even if they were only remotely blood related. Because of the flat societal organization and the principle that there are only close relatives I believe the European clan system does not fit Ojibwa society. See Appendix 1 for a visual chart of the two systems.

Families were expected to be responsible for visiting members of the same totem; even if they were strangers; the visitors would be treated as brothers or sisters and provided with both food and shelter. Totems were inherited and could not be changed. They were patrilineal so the children of the marriage would carry their father's totem. But the mother kept her totem.

There were totems of objects other than animals. One such example is my own totem. My father writes of his father, Out

On The Plain "... my father's totem is oak."[13] Out On The Plain's grandfather Little Thunder, both a war chief and a civil chief, signed several American treaties including the Peace Treaty of Greenville, the Treaty of Detroit and several British treaties including Treaties 6, 7 and 29. Invariably researchers have interpreted his totem as "an antler totem" or "caribou". But, his mark represented a tree, the mighty oak (see figure 1). Also, one of the signatories of Treaty 20 was "Pininse, of the White Oak Tribe".[14] These are examples of totems of trees. Trigger and Day mention a "Birch bark" totem as well.[15] Some other examples are a notched arrow of the Iliniouek, a big stone or rock of the Assinipoëls and the Flatheads had a vessel as a totem.[16]

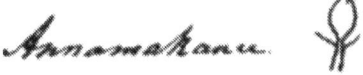

From Surrender #7 (1796). PAC, RG10, Vol. 1840, IT 027.

Figure 1—Oak Totem

Each individual had a personal name. An elder of the band usually named the child during a naming ceremony. More often

---

[13] Nicholas Plain, *The History of Chippewas of Sarnia and the History of Sarnia Reserve.* (Sarnia, ON: Privately Printed, 1951), 4.

[14] *Indian Treaties and Surrenders*, Treaty No. 20, vol. 1 (Toronto: Coles Publishing Company, 1992), 48.

[15] Bruce G. Trigger and Gordon M. Day, Southern Algonquin Middlemen, *Aboriginal Ontario*, (Toronto: Dundurn Press, 1994), 144.

[16] Extracts from an enumeration given by an unknown person, dated 12 October 1736 transcribed from NYCD, 1052-1058 in WHS, vol. 17, 245-252.

than not personal names are based on a dream, vision or an event and may not be given for up to two years. A personal name could be changed. For example a man might wish to honour his late father and so take his name for himself. Personal names were not used as signatory devices or in introductions. In fact during everyday communications a nickname, usually given during the person's youth, was preferred.

First Nations societies were oral societies. Because we had no written language we used wampum to seal treaties and other agreements. Wampum was usually a belt of beads with designs or pictograms on them but could be other objects such as a calumet, strings of beads, or an animal pelt. A speaker in council would hold up the wampum explaining what it represented and the acceptance of this wampum by the other party constituted a contract that remained in force until the wampum was surrendered to the party giving it. These contracts were held in the highest esteem and never broken, as it would have been a highly dishonourable thing to break one's word. Sir Francis Bond Head understood this truth and confirmed it in correspondence written by him to Lord Glenelg regarding his removal policy and dated 20th November 1836.

> It will be asked, in what way were these promises made; – it is difficult to reply to this question, as it involves the character of the Indian race.

> An Indian's word, when it is formally pledged, is one of the strongest moral securities upon earth: like the rainbow, it beams unbroken, when all beneath is threatened with annihilation.

> The most solemn form in which an Indian pledges his word is by the delivery of a wampum belt of shells and

when the purport of this symbol is once declared, it is remembered and handed down from father to son with an accuracy and retention of memory which is quite extraordinary.[17]

The Iroquois War ended with the Great Peace Treaty signed in Montreal in 1701. The Five Nation Confederacy secured a further peace with the Three Fires Confederacy at a council held at Lake Superior by delivering a wampum belt. Each generation was charged with renewing the peace by taking out the belt at a council and remembering the meaning of its symbols. In 1840 Ahnishenahbek chief Yellowhead read the belt at Renewal Council, which was attended by the Iroquois. See Yellowhead's speech in appendix 2 for a description of the belt and the meaning of its symbols.

After the Royal Proclamation of 1763 some 1500 First Nations chiefs and warriors including those of Aamjiwnaang met with Sir William Johnson at Niagara Falls. The purpose of the council was to secure a peace after Pontiac's War. They met in July 1764 and Johnson presented the First Nations with two wampum belts. On the first belt (see fig. 2) he said, "My children, I clothe your land, you see that Wampum before me, the body of my words, in this spirit of my words shall remain, it shall never be removed, this will be your Mat the eastern Corner of which I myself will occupy, the Indians being my adopted children their life shall never sink in poverty."

---

[17] *Report of the Indians of Upper Canada by a Sub-Committee* printed for The Aborigines Protection Society (London: William Ball, 1839), 20 available from
http://www.canadiana.org/ECO/SearchResults?id=14d4d351b2f38d44&query=Report+of+the+Indians+of+Upper&range=title&bool=all&subset=eng&pubfrom=&pubto= last accessed on 20 July 2006.

By these words he was coveting with the First Nations that the British recognized our ownership of the land and that they would respect that by only occupying the eastern corner of it leaving the rest for the First Nations to prosper in as allies.

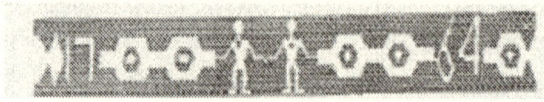

Figure 2—1764 Wampum

The second wampum presented by Johnson was called the twenty-four-nation belt (see fig. 3). The twenty-four figures represented the twenty-four First Nations of the covenant pulling a British ship laden with presents. This wampum symbolized the following words of the British, "My children, see, this is my Canoe floating on the other side of the Great Waters, it shall never be exhausted but always full of the necessities of life for you my Children as long as the world shall last. Should it happen anytime after this that you find the strength of your life reduced, your Indian Tribes must take hold of the Vessel and pull, it shall be all in you power to pull towards you this my Canoe, and where you have brought it over to this Land on which you stand, I will open my hand as it were, and you will find yourselves supplied with plenty." [18]

Unfortunately, although the Europeans understood the

---

[18] Darlene Johnston, Connecting *People to Place: Great Lakes Aboriginal History in Cultural Context*, prepared for The Ipperwash Inquiry, 14,15 available from http://www.ipperwashinquiry.ca/ last accessed on 20 July 2006.

solemness of wampum they did not follow through, as their words did not last.

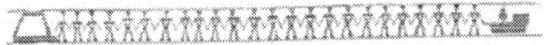

Figure 3—Twenty-Four Nation Wampum

2

Social Life

Gatherings, Games and Stories

During the summer months and into early autumn traditional gatherings took place. These were huge gatherings lasting for days and were held at traditional gathering places like Bawitig (Sault Ste. Marie) or at the mouth of the Black River. Great quantities of fish, berries and meat were consumed at these gatherings and drumming and dancing were constant. Games were played not just for entertainment but also for wagering. Old acquaintances were renewed as well as military alliances. These gatherings served to strengthen the Ahnishenahbek people keeping us one of the most powerful First Nations in the great lakes basin.

Some of the games we played were games of chance such as the game of straws and a game of dice. These games were played between villages or bands and some had been known to wager everything the village owned only to lose it all. Even so these losses never contributed to any animosity between opponents. Also, foot races were conducted throughout the gathering and were esteemed by all. Bougainville describes footraces being held at Detroit in 1757, "At Détroit foot races between the savages and the Canadians are as celebrated as horse races in England. They take place in the spring. Ordinarily there are live [sic] hundred savages present, sometimes as many, as fifteen hundred. The course is a half league, going and returning from Détroit to the village of the Poutéouatamis; the road is well made and wide. There are posts planted at the two extremities; the wagers are very considerable, and consist of packages of peltries laid against French merchandise such as is in use among the savages.[19]

We also played a ball game called baagaadowe, which the French called lacrosse. Sabrevois describes the game of lacrosse as follows:

> In summer they Play a great deal at la crosse, twenty or more on each side. Their bat [crosse] is a sort of small racket, and The ball with which they Play Is of very Heavy wood, a little larger than the balls we use in Tennis. When they Play, they Are entirely naked; they have only a breech-clout, and Shoes of deer-skin. Their bodies are painted all over with all Kinds of colors. There are some who paint their bodies with white clay, applying it to resemble silver lace sewed on all the seams of a coat; and, at a distance, one would take it for silver lace. They play for large Stuns, and often The prize Amounts to more than 800 Livres.

---

[19] 1757: Memoir of Bougainville translated from Pierre Margry, Relations et Memoires Inédits (Paris: 1867), 39-84 WHS, Vol. 18, 194.

They set up two goals and begin Their game midway between; one party drives The ball one way, and the other in the opposite direction, and those who can drive It to the goal are the winners. All this is very diverting and interesting to behold. Often one Village Plays against another, the poux against the outaouacs or the hurons, for very considerable prizes.[20]

The game of straws was described by Charlevoix as follows: " ...the game was played in the cabbin of the chiefs, and in a sort of square over against it. These straws are small rushed of the thickness of a stalk of wheat and two fingers in length. They take up a parcel of these in their hand, which generally consists of two hundred and one, and always of an unequal number. After they have well stirred them, and making a thousand contortions of body and invoking the genii, they divide them, with a kind of awl or sharp bone into parcels of ten: each takes one at a venture, and he to whom the parcel with eleven in it falls gains a certain number of points according to the agreement; sixty or four score make a party."[21]

The game of dice is also described by Sabrevois as follows: "This dish game is as follows. Eight little balls, red or black on one side, and yellow or white on the other, are tossed on a dish. When he who has the dish tosses them so that seven of the

---

[20] 1718: *Memoir on the Savages of Canada as far as the Mississippi River, Describing their Customs and Trade*, WHS, Vol. 16, 366-67. For full description of lacrosse, see *Jesuit Relations*, 10, 185-187, 231, 326-328; xv, 179.

[21] P. de Charlevoix in: *Journal of a Voyage to North America*, vol. 2 (London: Printed for R. and J. Dodsley 1761), 102 available from http://www.canadiana.org/eco/english/index.html last accessed 20 July 2006.

same color turn up, or all eight, he wins, and continues to play as long as he throws in this way; but when he throws otherwise, he or she with whom be Plays takes The dish and Plays in turn. In all these games they Play for large sums."[22]

Ahnishenahbek society was an oral society and as such produces great stories and storytellers. Most of the stories were designed to teach some truth or moral and were used as a form of entertainment. Each village had an official storyteller called debajehmujig who would entertain the whole community around a communal fire in the centre of the village during the warm summer months. During the winter these stories were used to pass the long winter evenings.

Our Ahnishenahbek ancestors would spend these evenings in the warm, cozy lodges with the adults entertaining all with traditional stories. There were hundreds of stories and in most the central character was Nanabozho. He was a being whose father was a mahnedoo or spirit being and his mother was human. He was a caricature of human nature and often he would not do the things he should or would do the things he should not. His character was flawed with the more base human characteristics. He would often stumble along in an almost comical way exhibiting the inner weakness that all human beings struggle with. He means well but his tendency to give into this inner weakness often turns his adventures into misadventures and his successes into failures. Some of the stories of Nanabozho were very long but most were short. The following is an example of one of these types of stories.

One day Nanabozho was walking in the woods when he came to a small lake. He spotted a flock of geese in the water and being hungry he thought one

---

[22] 1718: *Memoir*, WHS. Vol. 16, 369.

would make a good meal. But then he got greedy and thought he would like to cook and eat them all. He devised a plan to capture all the geese at once. He fashioned a long rope of elm bark and crept up to the water's edge. Slipping into the lake he swam up underwater, rope in hand, to the floating geese. He began tying the geese's feet together with the rope and when he had them all tied together he rose out of the water with a shout. The startled geese took off flying higher and higher with Nanabozho dangling from the end of the rope.

Finally his strength ran out and he let go of the rope while flying over woodland. He fell into a hollow tree where a bear was sleeping so he asked the bear to take him down out of the tree, which he did. His weight had pulled the flock of geese into the shape of a V and geese have been flying that way ever since.

Another example is the story about the little boy that was orphaned and had to live with his grandmother. Unfortunately his grandmother was of a wicked nature and soon began to torment the little boy so he wished Nanabozho would turn him into a bird. Nanabozho granted him his wish and he flew up into a tree that was growing near the old woman's wigwam. He started to laugh and his grandmother begged him to come back but he would not. And so we still have the red-breasted robin hanging around near people's lodges.

Shelter

In warm weather the cone shaped tepee was used and not a

great deal of attention was paid to its construction. Several straight saplings were cut about twelve feet long and about 2 inches in diameter at the butt end and 1 inch at the tip. Twelve poles would make a tepee of about ten feet in diameter. Two of these were fixed firmly in the ground, then crossed at a height of about six feet where they were tied with strips of basswood bark. A third pole was then leaned on the other two where they crossed and it was also tied securely. After this the rest of the poles were laid on the cross of the structure sloping to the ground and cedar bark was laid upon the framework leaving a hole at the top to let out any smoke from cooking fires that may have to be used during inclement weather. This was a temporary dwelling used only for sleeping and as shelter from gentle summer rains. At night a fire was built in the centre of the tepee in a smudge pot with green wood and leaves to make smoke. The hole at the top could be closed off with a piece of bark if need be. The smoke rose in the tepee leaving about two feet clear on the floor where we slept. The purpose of the smoke was to ward off mosquitoes.

During the winter months more attention was given to the construction of the wigwam. It was dome shaped and its footprint was either circular or oblong. Poles similar to the wigwam poles, but about 1½ inch in diameter at the butt end, were cut and planted into the ground 1 foot deep and eighteen inches apart. Enough poles were cut to encircle the base, which was about twelve feet in diameter. This size would have housed a family of two. The vertical poles were then bent inward toward the centre and tied. Cross poles were then tied to the sides for support. They could be smaller than the vertical poles about 1 inch at the butt end. The butt end was tied first and worked toward the tip. They were tied approximately 2 feet apart up to the top. A hole was left for the doorway, which could be closed off by hanging a blanket over it or with birch bark pinned to a frame. If the shape was oblong then a doorway was left at each end. The door was about 6 inches bigger than the opening all the way around. A smoke hole was left in the very centre of the top. The covering was pinned with large thorns. The wigwams were insulated first with woven mats, then cedar boughs and earth and finally covered with snow.

Bunks were built along the sides about eighteen inches high to sit or sleep on. Two-inch poles with forks at the top end were used for vertical posts tying the horizontal poles to the forks. Sticks ½ inch to ¾ inch were tied to the horizontal side rails for the bed. Cedar boughs were spread on top of the sticks for comfort.

A fire pit was made in the centre of the wigwam by laying large stones in a rectangle about 1 ½ foot wide by 2 foot long. The stones were buried half way in the ground. Two poles about 3 ½ feet long were planted a foot deep at each end of the pit. These had a fork on the top end to lay a pole across for cooking. Fresh meat or fish was laid over the cooking pole. Utensils such as brooms and birch bark or reed baskets and were made for use around the wigwam.

The wigwam was very warm and comfortable even in the coldest of winter nights as reported by Major Strickland in the mid nineteenth century. "The Indian wigwams are very warm. I have slept in them in the coldest weather with only one blanket wrapped about me, without experiencing the least inconvenience arising from either draft or cold.[23]

---

[23] Major C.M. Strickland, *Twenty-seven Years in Canada West or The Experience of an Early Settler*, ed. Agnes Strickland, Volume 2 (London: Richard Bentley Publisher, 1853), 34 available from

http://www.canadiana.org/eco/english/index.html last accessed 20 July 2006.

3

Economic Life

Agriculture and Gathering

The Ahnishenahbek did not engage in a lot of agriculture. Small garden plots were cultivated during the summer months when the band was congregated at the main village. It fell to the women and children to tend these gardens. Indian corn and pumpkin were the main crops and were only grown to supplement the band's food supply. Most of the foodstuffs were hunted, fished or gathered. The following are some of the fruits and nuts we gathered and how we processed them. This work also fell to the women and children.

Wild plums were gathered in October. They were plentiful and grew mainly along the shoreline of rivers and small lakes. Some of this crop was boiled with sugar and would fill the air with a light forest aroma. Sometimes they would be dried but mostly they would be boiled with maple sugar and made into a kind of cake dough. The plums would be boiled in a pot and stirred until the mass became thick, then spread out on a piece of hide or birch bark to the thickness of about one inch and dried in the sun. Once dry it forms a tough solid substance and it is rolled up and stored in birch bark boxes. They are stored in a hole in the ground, covered with earth and stored for the winter. During the winter months if there was no fresh meat, pieces of this substance were cut off and boiled with dried meat. Taking a couple of handfuls of shredded, dried meat and some wild plumbs and blueberries and boiling the mixture made venison soup.

No salt was used in traditional cooking. Maple sugar was used in preparing our meat as well as being sprinkled over fish boiled in water. Maple sugar was also used as a treat, which our children loved to eat piece by piece.

The wild cherry was also very common. Commonly called "sand cherries" they ripen in August. The women collected them at the same time as the blueberries and were prepared in various ways. One way was to crush the cherries between two rocks then mixing them with the fat of the deer and boiling the mixture until it forms dough. This was stored in birch bark boxes as a winter supply. Small red apples were also harvested from the wild apple trees dried and eaten as a desert.

Blueberries and black berries were also gathered and highly prized as a crop. They were usually dried by laying them out on frames of white wood and hung over a slow fire. When quite dry they were packed in birch bark boxes and later mixed with the bread dough. The sweet tasting berries were also boiled with fish or meat and would substitute for sugar late in the winter season if the sugar ran out.

Another berry of great value to us was the wild cranberry. They were bittersweet tasting berries yet pleasant and refreshing. They grew in swampy areas and ripened in October. These berries did not require drying, as they would last the whole winter without spoiling.

Wild hazelnuts were also collected and kept in bags. They

were used in place of butter often being eaten with their bread. Pounded nuts would also give the unsalted corn bread a delicious flavour. When there was neither nuts nor fat to take off the blandness of the corn bread a decoction of ashes was used. Warm water would be poured over the ashes from a very white wood. The course part would fall to the bottom. Then the ash water would be filtered and the ash water would be poured on the dough. This ash water was also using in making soup. Indian corn was also soaked in the water as part of its preparation process.

One of the roots we used for food was known as the swan potato. These grew in the water, on the banks of rivers and lakes. They were gathered and threaded on strings of white wood and then hung to in the lodge to be smoked. They were very small when dried, but swelled out when boiled. They were considered better than regular potatoes, very sweet and soft. Another root highly prized was the spruce root. It was a long, thin, knotty root light brown in colour, which was boiled and tasted like watercress. They were also dried and pounded between two stones into powder, which was used like flour to make bread. This powder could also be used to make soup by making a thin broth and adding any edible grain or pea or bean to it. Wild carrots were also boiled as a vegetable and tasted like the domestic carrot only stronger.

Several fresh herbs were also gathered and eaten fresh. One such herb used in cooking was the trout herb. The leaves were collected in the spring when young and they were called the leaves of the trout. They were used to make a very tasty and nutritious green fish soup. Even the bones and offal of the fish were used. They were pounded between stones then boiled with the trout herbs.[24]

Hunting and Trapping Camps

One of our main sources of food was meat with the pelts being used for clothing and other items. After the traditional gathering was held in the fall our main villages broke up and individual families of up to three would strike out into our traditional hunting territories to set up hunting and trapping camps. Wigwams would be constructed in a place that offered both shelter from wind and snow and a good water supply. The men would set out each day hunting or tending trap lines and return each evening to the camp. The women would spend the day tending the camp, cooking and processing game.

Deer and bear were particularly plentiful in Aamjiwnaang territory. Before the introduction of fire arms there were four different ways of hunting big game. The first was with a snare. Rope made of wild hemp would be used to snare even large game such as deer. When the deer was snared about the neck the rope would tighten. The more the deer struggled the less it could because the rope, winding itself around the neck, would choke the prey. The first half of the day was spent setting snares and the second half was spent driving the deer into the area where the snares had been set.

The second way was to take sharp spikes of wood and drive them into the ground just past a log on the deer trail. The deer would be unable to see the spikes and when jumping over the log would fall upon them killing them by piercing them through.

---

[24] J.G. Kohl, *Kitchi-Gami, Wanderings Around Lake Superior* (London: Chapman and Hall, 1860). 318-22 available from http://www.canadiana.org/eco/english/index.html last accessed 21 July 2006.

The third way was to chase the deer with dogs. In the summer they would be chased into the water where they could easily be disposed of. In the winter they would be chased into deep snow where they would tire quickly.

The fourth way of hunting deer was with bow and arrow. Bows were made of sufficient strength to be able to shoot an arrow through the side of a deer with no difficulty. In summer the hunter would wait near the shoreline of a lake or river where deer often go to feed on grass. In winter he would wait just off a deer trail where he was able to kill his game from a distance of up to fifty paces. Bows were generally made of well-seasoned ironwood, red cedar or hickory. The sharp point of the arrow was made of either bone or shell carved with barbed ends. Black bears were also hunted with bow and arrow. They were easy game in winter as they could be found hibernating in dens or hollow logs. They were more numerous in years when fruit, berries and nuts were most plentiful.[25] These were the hunting methods we used before contact and the advent of guns.

Trapping became more prevalent after the fur trade and European iron traps were used. But we also engaged in trapping before the fur trade. Snares and wooden box traps were used to trap smaller game such as rabbit, beaver, otter, martin, fisher and lynx. Often a hollow log would be used and they were most efficient after a heavy snowfall because small game would have difficulty finding food. The back end of the trap would not be closed off with anything solid but with a net because the game liked to see where it was going. A trap door was fixed to the top

---

[25] George Copway, *Indian Life and Indian History by an Indian Author* (Boston: Albert Colby and Co., 1858), 34-35, 37 available from http://www.canadiana.org/eco/english/index.html last accessed 21 July 2006.

of the log with leather hinges. A hole was also made in the top of the log. A cord was run from the door to a trigger inside the log. It would hold the trap door at a 45° angle from the ground. The trigger would be attached to the inside of the log about 2 inches off the floor. It would be a piece of flat wood about 6 inches long and 2 inches wide. This trigger would be notched at its midpoint, as would the side of the log. A catch, stick about 6 inches long, would also be notched at its midpoint and the cord would be tied taut at the notch. This catch would be placed in the notches on the trigger and the inside of the log. Corn or some dried fruit would be attached to the trigger. The weight of the animal on the trigger would release the catch and the weight of the trap door would cause it to fall closing the open end of the log.

Instead of using a log sometimes a box would be constructed of 1 inch saplings notched and tied together. A large rock would be tied to the top of the box. One end of the box would be held up at 45° with a trigger device. This trigger was made of 3 sticks ½ inch in diameter notched and with the bark left on. It was made in a figure four shape with the bait end extending to the centre of the upheld box. When the bait end was disturbed the whole device collapsed allowing the box to fall over the animal trapping it. The heavy rock would hold the box over the trapped animal.

Sugar Camps

After wintering in small family hunting camps we would congregate at various sugar bushes in groups of six or so families. This gathering would take on an almost festival atmosphere as old acquaintances were renewed after a long and isolated winter. This would make the job of making maple syrup and sugar a very joyous occasion. The men would continue to hunt and the women and children would run the sugar camps.

A sugar boiling wigwam would be built in the same manner as the oblong wigwam described in the "Shelter" section above except the footprint of this wigwam would be about thirty feet long and sixteen feet wide. The fire pit would run the length of the structure and a hanging frame about 4 feet high would serve to hang the cooking kettles on. Copper kettles were used to boil the sap and the fires were tended continually. A smaller tepee type structure would also be erected in order to store the sugar making utensils. Wigwams were also constructed for the families to live in.

When the wigwams were ready the trees were tapped with spiles. This was done by first cutting a groove into the tree on the sunny side about 3 feet above the roots. The spiles were then pounded into the tree to a depth of approximately 3 inches and sealed with hot pitch. The spiles were made from elderberry stems with the pith pushed out, one end sharpened, and the other end notched to hold the sap pail. The pails were made of birch bark and folded at the bottom, not sewn. A small pail could fill up in an hour at the height of the season. These were collected in the morning and at night.

Toboggans were used to haul the buckets of sap back to the boiling wigwam. The toboggans were made of hardwood cut during the winter when the trees have no sap. The front end was heated by boiling and bent upwards. They were pulled from the front but had a rope tied to the back so one person could control any sliding downhill.

The sap was poured into the copper kettles and continuously boiled until evaporation left sweet syrup. It takes thirty to forty gallons of sap to boil down to one gallon of syrup. With more boiling and evaporation the syrup would crystallize leaving a solid maple sugar product. This crystallized sugar was the bulk of their product but just before crystallization some of the very thick syrup would be poured into wooden moulds where it would harden to make a sort of rock candy. A fourth sugar product was made by pouring some of the thick syrup into the snow to cool it very quickly. In this case the syrup would not crystallize but turn into a kind of taffy.[26] People would be assigned times to tend the fires and continually stir the kettles to prevent the sap from burning. This went on until the sap stopped running at which time the spiles were removed and the tree sealed with pitch. Utensils were stored in the storage tepee until next year and the group would move on to the fishing camps.

Since the hunting camps and the sugar bushes were far inland and too far to have carried our good canoes we would build temporary ones from the bark of elm trees. These were made entirely out of one roll of bark of the swamp-elm. It was a ruder canoe than the birch bark one described below as it was merely sewn up at both ends and the seams gummed. Two thwarts were then fastened to the upper edges of the canoe to keep it spread to a width of about 3½ feet. All of the produce from the hunt and the sugar camps were loaded into these temporary canoes and they were only used to descend the fast moving rivers that flowed into Lake Huron or the St. Clair. This also served to protect the good birch bark canoes as the white water rapids of rivers like the Aux Sable and Maitland could easily damage them.[27]

---

[26] Kohl., *Kitchi-Gami*, 323-24.

[27] Strickland, *Twenty-seven Years*, 49-50.

Fishing Camps

Many different kinds of fish were caught and in various ways. The rivers and streams provided brook trout, perch and bass. Lake Huron produced very large lake trout. Major Strickland was travelling on a schooner bound for Mackinaw in the early 1800's when met by nine canoes of Ahnishenahbek fishermen who came on board to barter. One of the passengers traded for a lake trout weighing "no less than seventy-two pounds".[28] Herring were also taken from the lake, but the sturgeon was a particular delicacy. One of the main staples of course was white fish. White fish was most plentiful and was so tasty it could be eaten quite regularly without becoming tiresome. Its meat was snow white and when boiled to perfection it became rather flaky but not dry. Some of our favourite fishing areas were in Lake Huron above the rapids of the St. Clair River, in the St. Clair itself and in Lake Huron at Kettle Point and at the mouth of the Aux Sable River.

We used various methods of fishing including spearing, netting, line and hook, and weirs. Spearing was extensively used. A pole 8 to 10 feet long and approximately 1½ inch in diameter at the butt end was used to make spears. The points were made from two pieces of ¼ inch iron rod twelve to fifteen inches long. A long point was filed on one end and a short end was filed the other end of each rod. One rod was about an inch longer that the other. The short points were bent at 90 degree angles about 3/8 of an inch long. A couple of barbs were cut in the rods with a cold chisel. The butt end of the spear was cut with a groove about six inches deep. The sharp ends of the rods would be forced into the groove with the barbs facing each other and the end of the spear wrapped with cord or rawhide.

---

[28] Ibid.,132-33.

The prongs would be tapered slightly outward.

Spearing was done in summer and winter as well as both day and night. At night torches were used. Sturgeons were speared in the winter on the ice. A hole was cut in the ice about 2 feet in diameter. A small hut of poles and animal hide was built over this hole and the fisherman would crawl into the hut face down with his head over the hole but leaving his legs outside. Daylight would light up the water beneath the transparent ice all around the hole and the artificial darkness produced by the hut and the fisherman's head prevented any reflection. The fisherman could see to a depth of forty feet watching for any fish swimming by. He could then thrust his spear at his unsuspecting prey.

Nets were used during the spring fish runs. Dip nets were fashioned by attaching a net about 2 feet long to a hoop and attaching the hoop to a long pole. Fishermen would then canoe out into the rapids at the mouth of the St. Clair River. With one standing in the canoe while the other steered he would dip for white fish all the while keeping his balance. One swoop of the net would catch 7 or 8 fish at a time, which would be deposited into the bottom of the canoe in one motion. When the canoe was full they would be dumped on the shore and the fishermen would return to the rapids. Only the Ahnishenahbek were known to fish in such a manner and with such a high degree of efficiency.

A lure was sometimes used when spearing the fish from an ice hole. It would be fashioned from a piece of wood or bone and sometimes dyed blue like a small herring. It would be tied to a line and weighted down with a piece of lead. Larger fish would then be enticed to the top of the water and when near enough to the opening would be speared.[29] Fish weirs were also built during the spawning runs, which would force them into the holding pens for harvesting.

The following is a description of how fish were traditionally dried:

> Pat and Rebecca Shewaybick and translator Roy Spence from Webikwe, Ontario, visited the Bay Mills Indian Community Gnoozhekaaning Cultural Center June 21-22, 2000. Webikwe is a small northern Ontario community of about 600 Ahnishenahbek who still follow the old ways. The Shewaybicks and their children often spend weeks in the woods hunting and gathering. They visited Bay Mills, on the Lake Superior shoreline about 20 miles west of the Soo Locks, to show the community there how to powder fish so it can be preserved without refrigeration. Whitefish provided by a tribal fisher was used for the lesson.

> The Shewaybick family also shared their traditional philosophy of life. According to Roy, it's up to them to look after each other and the land, and in this way they can preserve their way of life. Roy, a Webikwe council member, works hard to educate the Ontario government leaders about the Ahnishenahbek culture.

> First a tepee is put up to smoke the fish. Juniper boughs are then gathered and placed in the tepee to keep the dampness out. The fish are then prepared for smoking. The heads and spines are removed, but both fillets remain attached to the tail. The bones keep the flesh from falling apart during smoking. The

[29] Kohl, Kitchi-*Gami*, 325-31.

cleaned fish are then placed on drying sticks. The fish smoke with the sides held apart by the stick, to facilitate smoking. The smoked fish are pulled out of their skins and chunked into a heavy iron skillet to be powdered. The bones are kept in the mixture and fall apart much as canned salmon bones do, providing more nutrition. The fish is stirred back and forth over the heat, breaking it up more and more until it is completely dried and powdered, and ready to store.[30]

Trade

A report on the American Colonies to King George I written on the 8th of September 1721 stated that, "From the north east of the Lake Erie to a fort on the lake St. Clair, called fort Chartrim, [Pontchartrain] is about eight leagues sail; here the french have a settlement, and often 400 traders meet there along this Lake they proceed about seven leagues further, and thence to the great Lake Huron about ten leagues; hence they proceed to the straits of Michilimackinack 120 leagues. Here is a garrison of about 30 french, and a vast concourse of traders, sometimes not less than 1,000, besides Indians, being a common place of rendezvous. At and near this place the Outawas an Indian nation are settled."[31]

Undoubtedly the Ahnishenahbek of Aamjiwnaang would have traded at Detroit. We also wanted to trade at Albany with the British and we would travel that far if the goods were much

---

[30] A description complete with photos of powdering fish using traditional native methods is available from http://www.great-lakes.net/teach/history/native/native_9.html last accessed June 24, 2005.

[31] *Reports on American Colonies 1721*-1762, from the NAC in MPHSC, Vol. 19, 5.

cheaper. British goods were also known to be of better quality than French goods. In "An Abridgment of the Indian Affairs" on June 28th 1729 regarding trade with the far Indians it was reported "The Commissrs receive them very friendly & give them Assurances of Protection & good usage in Trade & tell them that they will find they can buy at Albany more for One Bever than for 3 with the French".[32]   Another manuscript reports:

> It must not be forgotten, also, that with very few exceptions the Indian tribes of the west remained faithful to the cause of France until the end of the French domination in America. Frontenac, Denonville, and other French officials had the same distrust of the Indians as Perrot; but the latter governor admitted that they were attracted to the English by the better market thus afforded for the sale of their peltries. As proof of this, is cited a Ms. dated 1689, in the archives of the Marine, showing the difference in prices at Orange [Albany] and Montreal; for one beaver-skin an Indian received at Orange forty pounds of lead, or a red blanket, or a large overcoat, or four shirts, or six pairs of hose, while at Montreal each of these items cost him two pelts, and even three for the above quantity of lead. A gun cost two pelts at Orange, and five at Montreal; and one pelt procured for the Indian eight pounds of gunpowder from the English, while the French demanded four for that quantity. "The other petty wares which the savages buy in trade from the French are given to them by the

---

[32] Wraxall, *Harvard Historical Studies,* vol. 21, 177, OVGLEA: MC 1723-1730.

English as part of the bargain. The English give six pots of brandy for one beaver-skin; this is rum, or guildive (otherwise sugar-cane brandy), which they import from the islands of America [i.e., the West Indies]. The French have not standard [of price] for the brandy trade; some give more, and others less, but they never go so high as one pot for one beaver-skin... It is to be noted that the English make no difference as regards the quality of the beaver-skins, which they buy all at the same price-- which is more than fifty per cent higher than the French give; and, besides, there is more than one hundred per cent difference in the value of their trade and that of ours-- Tailhan.[33]

The French did everything in their power to prevent any First Nations trade with the British. In 1724 the following was reported in An Abridgement of Indian Affairs made to the Governor of New York: "14 July Several Far Indians arrive to Trade with Bever &c & say the French used every Artifice in their Power to prevent their coming to Albany & had by promises & Threatenings prevailed upon 30 Canoes of Indians to go to Canada who had never been at Albany & intended to have come with them hither".[34] Far Indians were First Nations from the Upper Great Lakes, mostly Ahnishenahbek including the Mississauga.

This trade activity like most travel was done using the birch

---

[33] Emma Helen Blair, Memoir on the Manners, Customs and Religion of the Savages of North America as described by Nicolas Perrot, *The Indian Tribes of the Upper Mississippi Valley and Regions of the Great Lakes*, Volume 1 (Cleveland,: The Arthur H. Clark Co., 1911, n 181, 258.

[34] Wraxall, *Harvard Historical Studies*, vol. 21, 152, OVGLEA: MC 1723-1730.

bark canoe. This was a light, highly manoeuvrable vessel, yet it was extremely strong and able to carry very heavy loads. They were made of various lengths from fourteen feet for a family to thirty feet for trading or war. We constructed them in the following manner.

First the proper tree was selected. It was as large and smooth as possible to provide the largest sheets of bark. The larger the sheets the less sewing required. It should also have been free of any lichen growth, which may allow the bark to split under pressure. Also not forked at the top. Ideally a single piece was needed the length of the canoe and wide enough to reach the gunwales at the centre of the canoe. Otherwise pieces would have to be sown on to the sides in order to reach the gunwales. This piecing would have required double stitching.

The tree was either felled or the bark taken from the tree while standing. Two incisions were made around the tree at each end then one vertical cut was made from top to bottom. The taking of the bark had to be done at the proper time of year, sometime in June. If the air temperatures were right the bark would pop off.

The construction site was chosen and a flat bed of sand free of rocks or twigs was spread out in a rectangular shape. A wigwam was built over the site to prevent any direct sunlight from drying out the materials too quickly and curling the bark. The bottom piece was spread out on the bed of sand with the outside or white side facing up. An oblong shaped wooden canoe form with pointed ends was then placed on the bottom piece. The sides were then drawn up the length of the canoe and cedar steaks were driven into the ground along both sides of the canoe to enable the canoe to begin to take form. The ends of the piece of bark were then pinched together and held by cedar pins. The outer steaks were then tied together with strips of basswood bark. If the sides of the bark were not sufficient to reach the whole length of the gunwales then strips of bark needed to be double stitched onto the sides. Four long thin cedar gunwales were then put in place along the perimeter of the canoe two on each with the bark in between. The inner gunwales would have already been mortised to receive the three thwarts. These would keep the canoe from spreading. Once in place the gunwales were lashed together the full length of each side of the canoe.

The bow and stern were worked on next. Stems were made from cedar pieces about 1¾ inch wide 5/8 of an inch deep and 27 inches long. They would be split so the rings were running across the flatter part of the wood. Each stem piece was then split with a knife into 8 pieces for easier bending. The stems were bent into the proper shape by pouring boiling water over them to make them pliable, bending them into shape and tying them with basswood bark string so they would hold their shape. When dried they were placed inside the bow and stern and pegged temporarily into place. The gunwales were lashed together and the excess bark was then trimmed and sewn together. Either tamarack or cedar roots were used in the sewing.

Now the cedar ribs were bent into shape. They were soaked for several days in water to make them pliable and when they were to be shaped, boiling water was poured over them to make them even more pliable. About forty were cut about ½ inch thick and 2 inches wide for a fourteen-foot family canoe. While standing on them one at a time the ends were gradually pulled up until the proper bend was achieved. They were then inserted into the canoe in their proper place and left for a day to dry. They were then removed and cedar planking, pieces about 1/8 of an inch thick and 3 to 4 inches wide were laid on the bottom of the canoe for flooring. The flooring was held into place by reinserting the ribs. A gunwale cap was then installed and held in place by birch wood pegs to protect the lashing holding the gunwales together.

The canoe was then inverted for pitching. Pitch was made from spruce gum and deer tallow. The canoe was sealed with this mixture wherever the bark had been cut and sewn. A container of this pitch was carried by the canoeist for use in repairing during travel. Once the pitch was dry the canoe was ready for use. It would take three to five weeks to build a canoe taking into consideration the time to find the right tree and to prepare the site and paraphernalia needed for construction.

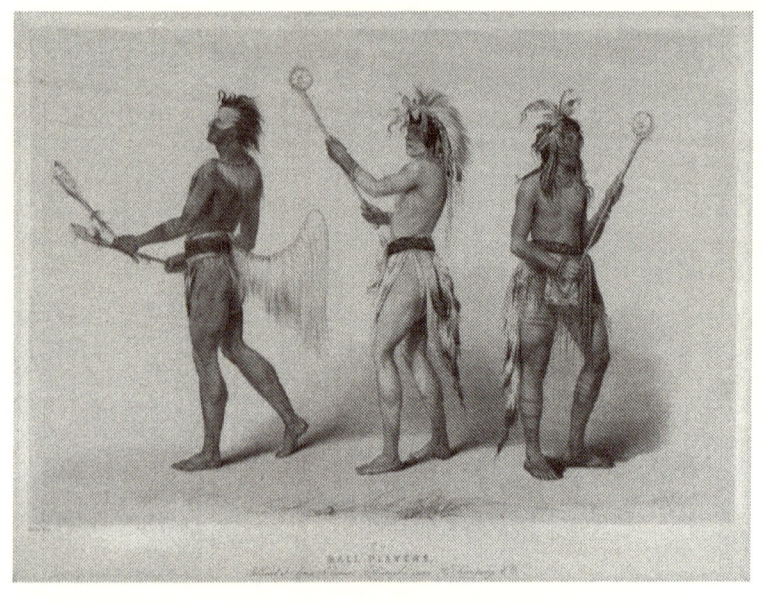

Baagaadowe or playing the game of lacrosse. These players were sketched by George Catlin in the 1800's.

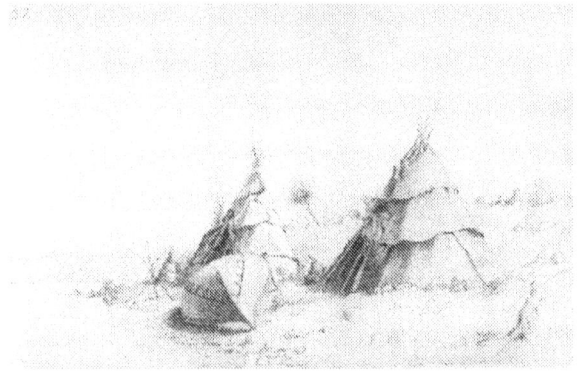

Ojibwa tepees on Lake Huron, on the shores of
Georgian Bay.

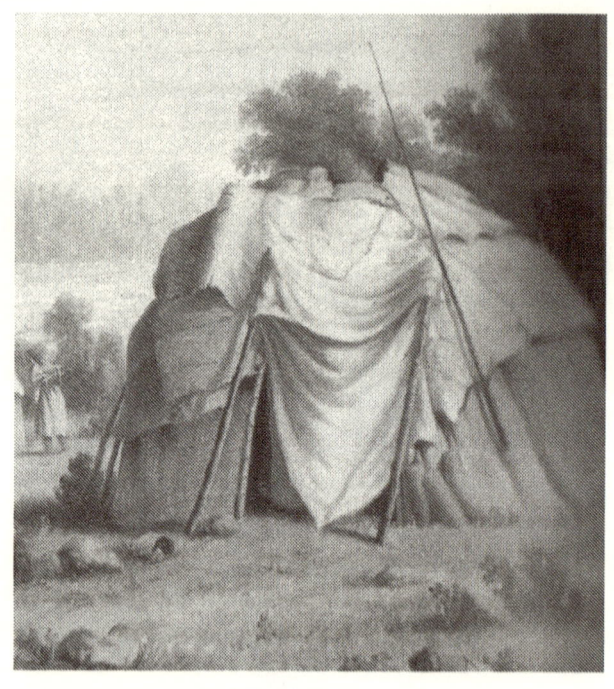

Ojibwa wigwam. Detail from a painting (1846) by
Paul Kane of an Ojibwa village at Sault Ste. Marie.

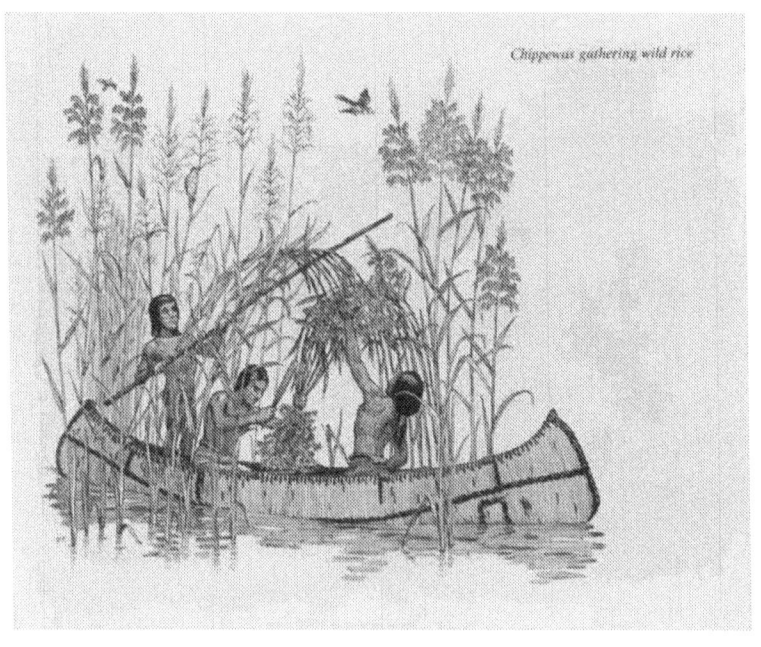

Illustration of three Chippewas gathering wild rice in a canoe.
Courtesy of WHS.

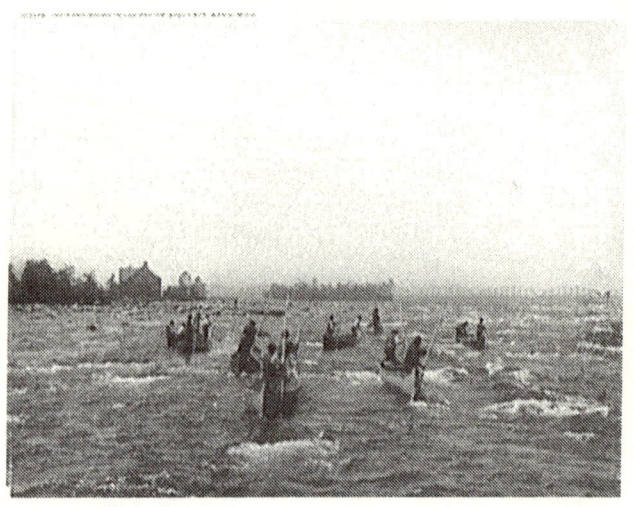

Fishing ca 1900 on the St. Marys River.

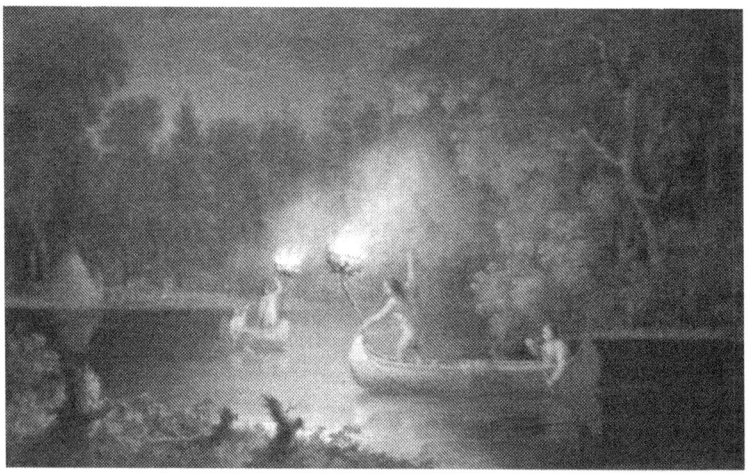

Spearing Salmon by Torchlight, an oil painting by Paul Kane depicting Menominees spear fishing at night by torchlight and canoe on the Fox River. Ahnishenahbek fishers used the same method as their Menominee brothers.

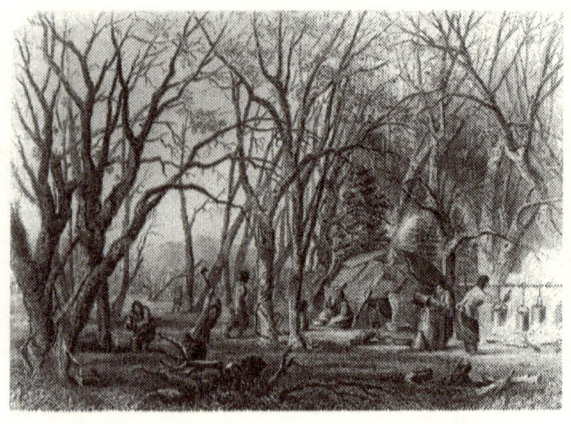

Drawing of an Ahnishenahbek sugar camp ca. 1850. Courtesy WHS.

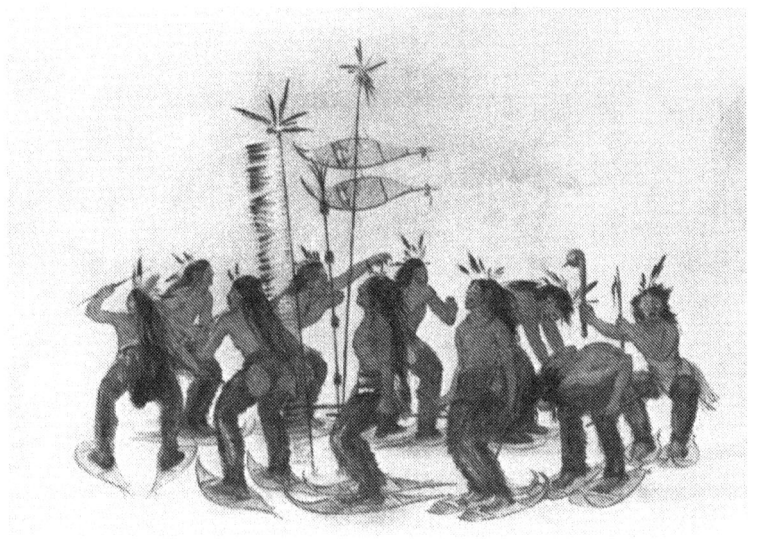

The Snowshoe Dance by George Catlin 1835. Ahnishenahbek traditional dance performed at the first snowfall.

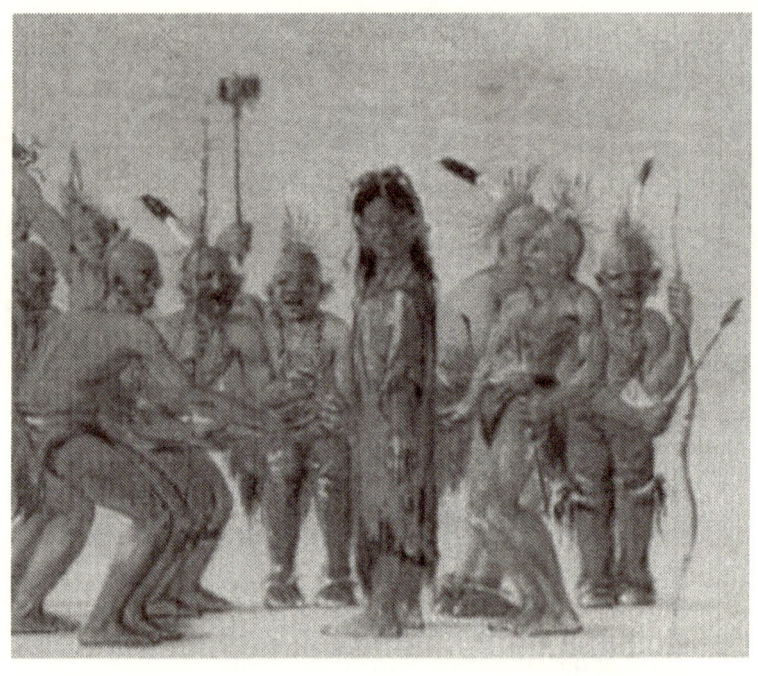

"Dance to the Berdache" by George Catlin. Drawn on the Great Plains among the Fox and Sac. This sketch depicts a ceremonial dance to celebrate the two-spirit person.

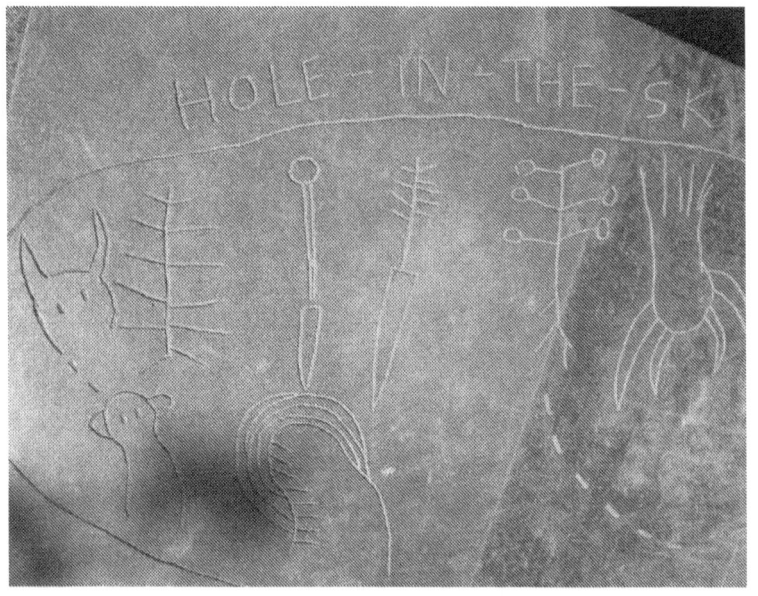

Hole in the Sky, 1981, Andrew Dutkewych. A section of Top
Carvings held at the Art Gallery of Algoma, Sault Ste. Marie,
Canada.

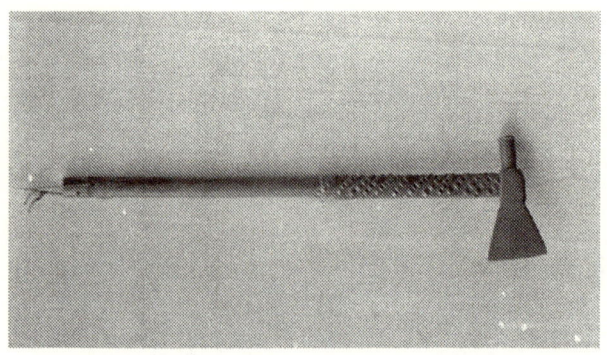

Pipe Tomahawk photo by D. F. Barry , between 1854-1930.

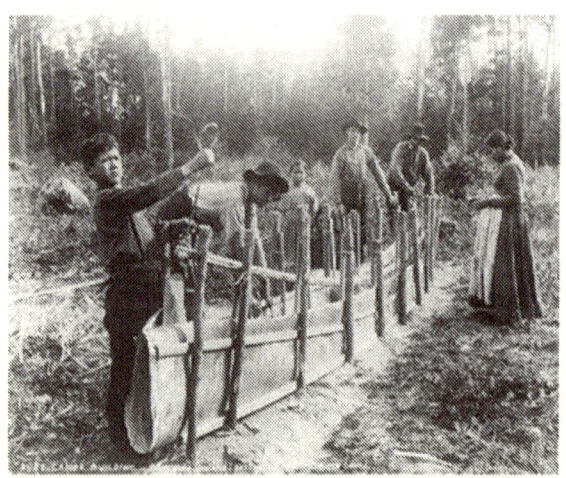

Building birch canoes, c.1895.
Courtesy Minnesota Historical Society

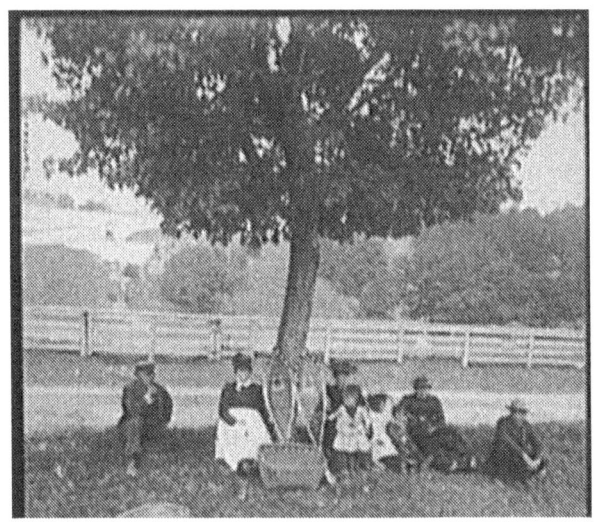

Basket Selling ca 1900 on Manitoulin Island.

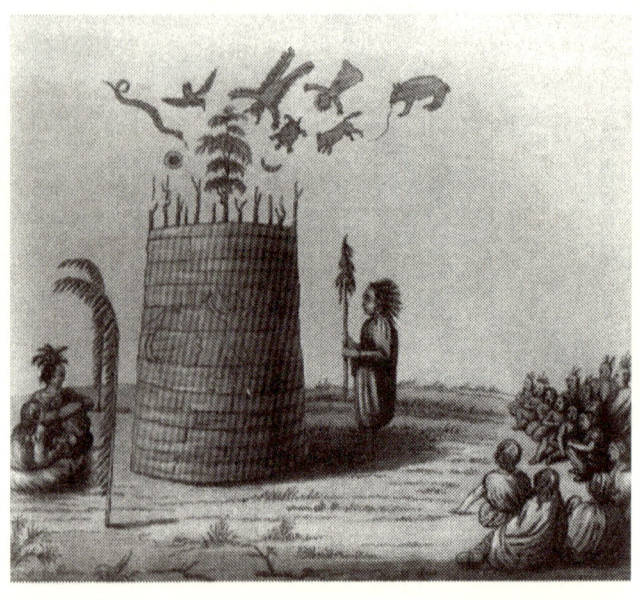

Drawing of a shaking tent used by Ahnishenahbek conjurers to converse with the spirits. The cedar pole with the branches still on acts as a conduit and the various animals above it represent the spirits entering the tent.

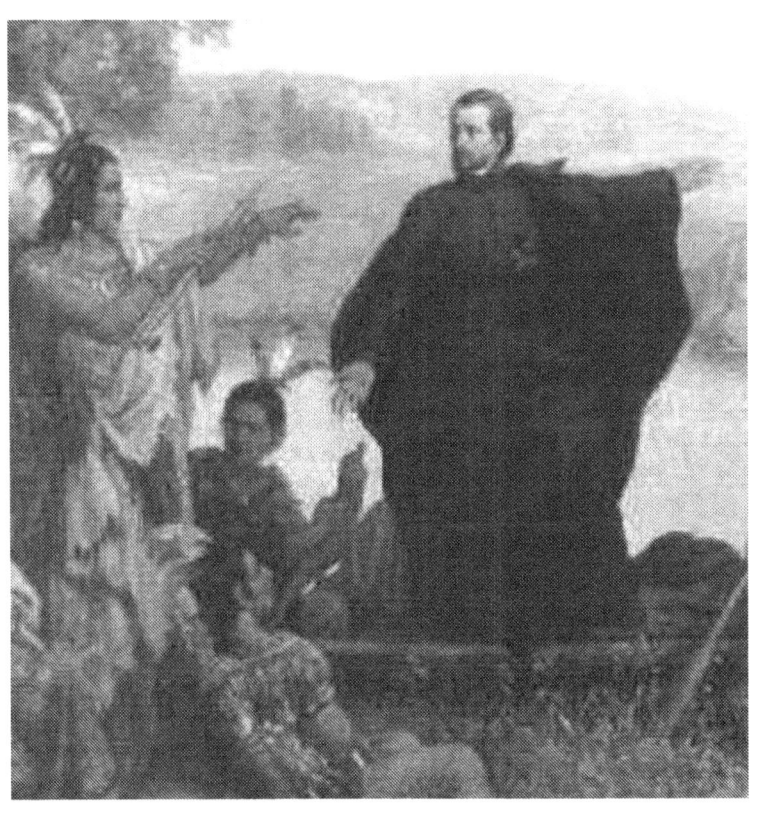

Father Jacques Marque (Jesuit Missionary 1637-1675.)
preaching.

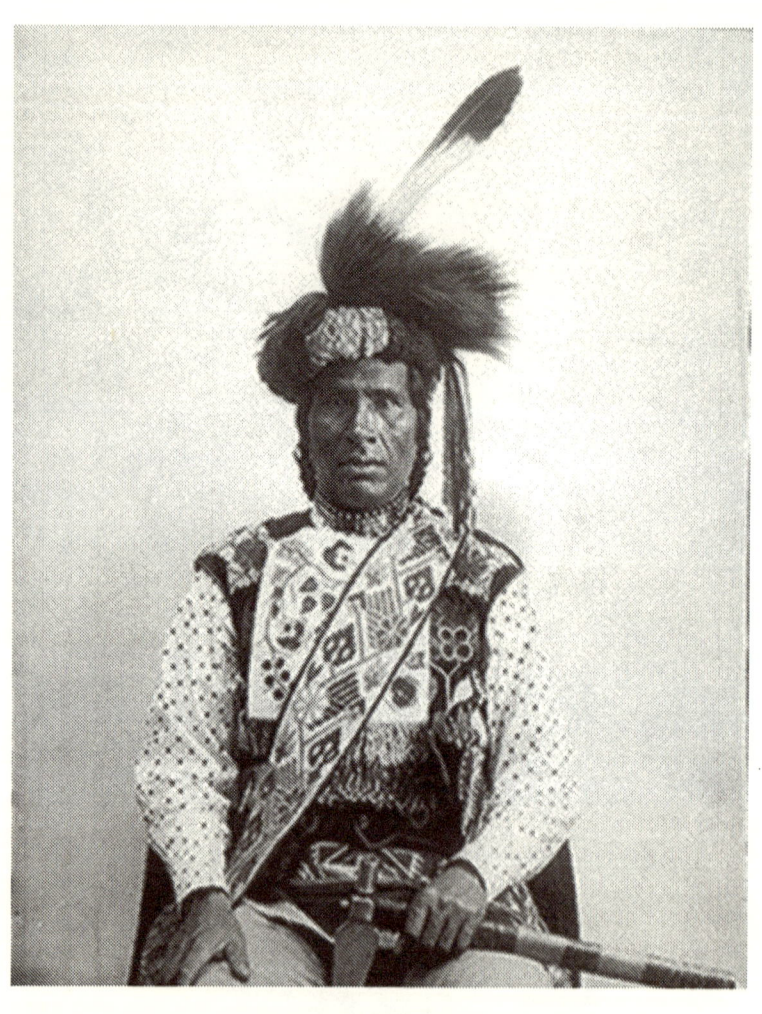

One-Called-From-A-Distance (Midéwiwin), an Ahnishenahbi
from Minnesota, 1894.

4

Religious Life

Beliefs

The Ahnishenahbek world was both a corporeal and a spiritual world at once. Our daily lives were inspired by the interaction of spiritual beings that affected the everyday activities of our physical world. A spirit being commonly called a manitou is more properly called a muneedoo, although the meaning of the word is not limited to spirit. It can also refer to the essence, characteristic or power of a thing such as a plant or a ceremony. Needless to say this caused much confusion for the early Christian missionaries. Of these spiritual beings there was one overall and creator of all. This spirit being was known as Kitchi-Muneedoo or the Great Mystery.

Kitchi-Muneedoo was transcendental, unknowable and therefore shrouded in mystery. However, we believed that he was the creator of all things including the other muneedoog. In the creation story Kitchi-Muneedoo created the heavenly expanse, in which he place the sun and moon and a myriad of stars. He created the earth and all that is in it, the rivers and lakes, plants and trees, birds, fish and animals all according to his vision. He also created the Ahnishenahbek or the real people. He also created the spiritual realm and all the muneedoog according to the purpose of his vision. One of these kinds of muneedoog were personal spirit beings and their purpose was to act as a guide and helper in the Ahnishenahbi's life as well an intercessor between the person and Kitchi-Muneedoo.

This creation story demonstrates a belief in God and an understanding of the origin of things. It also served as an example for the Ahnishenahbek to follow and so the tradition of seeking their personal muneedoog through a vision or dream was developed. In this tradition a young person of puberty or adolescent age would prepare himself for his vision quest by purifying himself in the sweat lodge ceremony. When this was completed he would seek out a place to meditate in the wilds preferably a high place where the wind was constant. There he would fast and meditate until his vision came. This vision would always contain a central figure represented by an animal, bird, reptile or some other creature and this would be his personal muneedoo. This muneedoo would have the characteristics of its corporeal representation and would use them in his interaction with the individual. This personal muneedoo would be a patron to his assigned person for life.

This ritual was available to either sex but the participants were almost exclusively young men.

Most muneedoog were good most of the time but could at times be mischievous or even spiteful. A good example of this type of muneedoo was the Mamagwasewug or the hidden or covered beings. They were little spirit beings commonly called fairies or sprites. The preferred to live along riverbanks or wetlands and are at most times invisible. Some of the old ones say they have seen them and have even talked to them. They are described as two to three feet tall, have a human form walking erect but their faces are covered with soft hair. They are said to be fond of shooting firearms and love bright bits of cloth. If one helps them to attain these things one will be rewarded with long life or success in hunting. The following is a story of a group of Mamagwasewug living along the St. Clair River in the 1820s.

In 1824 a Scottish family who were living on the banks of the St. Clair River came under harassment by some invisible entities. Their property was being assailed; first their poultry suffered seizures and died then their livestock. Next the house was attacked. Small pieces of lead and stones were thrown at the windows, which broke and they landed on the floor. Later, live coals were found placed in different parts of the house and at first were discovered by the family and extinguished just in time. However, eventually the house burned down.

The family, friends and neighbours attributed these occurrences to witchcraft and a famed witch doctor from Niagara Falls named Troyer was called in. He attempted to exorcise the property by shooting off his gun, which he said was loaded with silver bullets. He said this was the only kind of weapon that would be effective against a witch. While this was going on the local magistrate heard of it and issued an arrest warrant for Mr. Troyer. He heard of the warrant and so beat a hasty retreat back to Niagara Falls.

Pazhekezhikquashkum, the old Otahwah head chief and shaman from Walpole Island was consulted and he confided that he knew what was going on all the time. He said the place on which the house stood was the former residence of the Mamagwasewug but when the Scotchman built his house on the spot where the Mamagwasewug lived they moved back into the poplar grove. They lived there for several years but then the Scotchman cleared and burnt the grove. This made the Mamagwasewug angry and feeling indignant at such treatment they exacted revenge on his property.[35]

Now some muneedoog were pure evil. The most evil of all of them was matchi-muneedoo or the evil spirit. He is often compared with Satan of the Judeo-Christian world. One of the evil muneedoog that we feared the most was the Windego. Our understanding of the relationship between the corporeal world and the spiritual realm allowed for crossover. An Ahnishenabi could become a spirit being. This explains the origin of the Windego.

The Windego was a giant. It towered over the average man being eight to ten feet tall and its long strides made it possible for it to outrun even the swiftest Ahnishenahbi. Its grey, putrid skin gave it a telltale rancid odour. It was pulled tight over its skeleton and its eyes were sunken giving it a grotesque appearance. This monster was a cannibal. It suffered from an insatiable hunger for human flesh. The more of it ate the hungrier it became. Its only objective was to try to satisfy its insatiable desire. Yet it was anaemic due to its perpetual starvation, as its food had no nutritional value.

---

[35] Jones, *History*, 157-159.

In Ahnishenahbek lore the Windego represented one of the more despicable of human traits, greed. Each individual in Ahnishenahbek society was expected to be giving toward the community in all areas. Sharing was required for the community to survive and if for example, winter supplies ran out and the people faced starvation then we all faced it together. Sometimes human greed would surface and an individual would horde to the detriment of others. This greedy person could suffer one of two fates. Either he or she could be turned into a Windego or be eaten by one. The following is an Ahnishenahbek legend about one person that became a Windego.

One particular summer drought had visited the territory of a certain Ahnishenahbek band. The berries did not ripen so there was no harvest and game became very scarce. The following winter hunters returned to their hunting camps empty-handed too many times. The people were reduced to eating roots and tree bark trying to survive.

One individual's thoughts turned from the survival of the group to his own. He decided to visit a shaman to ask him for a talisman that would enable him to find food for himself. The shaman gave him some powder made from certain plant roots and told him to make a tea of it. After he drank it in secret he would be able to find food for himself. So, he awoke the next morning before anyone else made the tea and drank it.

Surprisingly he immediately began to grow. Taller and taller until he was twice the height of an ordinary man. And such long strides he had. He could cover great distances in so short a time and he could outrun even the swiftest of deer. Over the hills his long strides carried him far away from his family's hunting camp. He reached the top of a certain hill where he could see a village belonging to a different band of Ahnishenahbek in a valley. He was so excited to see more prosperous people that he began to shout and run toward the village. However, his voice was deep and loud like the crack of thunder directly overhead. He was an awesome sight thundering and bounding down the hillside at twice the speed of a full-grown buck. The people of the village were so frightened that many of them dropped dead in their tracks. The others fled.

In next to no time he entered the village where there were plenty of provisions. He was famished but he had no craving for dried fruit, fish and venison. Instead the aroma of the dead bodies that lay strewn on the ground instilled in him an eerie desire for human flesh. He began to taste some and soon devoured a whole body. But it was not enough. He was still starving so he began to eat more of the dead people and the more he ate the hungrier he became. The tea along with his own selfish greed had turned him into a Windego!

Soon one of the village's most renowned warriors returned to the empty village. This warrior was filled with grief when he discovered what had happened but his grief soon turned to rage. With all of his people gone he had nothing left but revenge and he set out on the trail of the Windego. With great determination he soon overtook him. The Windego was in his habitual weakened state and begged for mercy but the warrior had none. In a rage he killed the Windego on the spot leaving his corpse as carrion for the vultures and crows.

Ahnishenahbek cultural lore was filled with stories of Windigos. Each community had their own but all had the same morals to teach about generosity, greed, moderation and excesses.

The Ahnishenahbek belief system revolved around a secret medicine society called the Midéwiwin Medicine Society or The Grand Medicine Society. Sometimes it was just referred to as

"The Lodge". It was secret only in the sense that the multitude of medicines used for curing and divining and each individual chant that went with them was knowledge acquired by lodge members only through a long and arduous training program. Individuals were usually chosen as young children or adolescents according to a natural ability seen in them. They then would be initiated as trainees in an initiation ceremony. When they became the age to seek their vision, if they were boys, they would then be assigned a tutor. Girls were not required to seek their vision although they could if they wished.   For an eyewitness account of a Midéwiwin initiation ceremony recorded by James Evans, Wesleyan missionary to the Ahnishenahbek of Aamjiwnaang see appendix 3.

There were four orders in the hierarchy of the Lodge called degrees. After an initiate went through his or her initial training, which would take a year they became a candidate for First Degree Midéwiwin shaman or priest. After purifying himself in a sweat lodge ceremony he would undergo another Midéwiwin ceremony held in a specially constructed lodge called the Medéwigun. It was built in the shape of a rectangle about 50 feet long by 25 feet wide facing east and west. It was open on the top and had a doorway at each end. A freshly cut cedar post called a Medéwitik stood inside the lodge and near it a fire would be built. This ceremony accepted the candidate as a First Degree shaman. As an accredited First Degree he would now have the right to paint one bar on his face and preside at funerals and Feast of the Dead. Sometime after the ceremony, when the candidate was ready, he had to declare his intention of seeking the next level before he could go on. These steps were repeated for each degree with some changes in the actual liturgy of each and in the privileges acquired by the candidates. After a member completed his Fourth Degree training and ceremony he was accredited as a Fourth Degree Midéwiwin Priest and would follow his vocation as either diviner or healer. He would still, however, have to attend one Midéwiwin ceremony each year for renewal.[36]

The spiritual realm and the physical realm were often connected through the practice of medicine. Medicine was not practiced as it is today. Medicine was a part of religion and it was the shaman that had the responsibility of serving his community with healing as well as communion with the spirit world. There were two types of shaman in the Midéwiwin Lodge, the healing shaman and the divining shaman. Sometimes these medicine men were called jugglers and conjurors respectively.

The healing shaman, called nanandawi, had a catalogue of cures for various ailments made up of the right mixtures of herbs and plants. Of course for the healing power to be released these mixtures had to be invoked with the right ceremonies and chants. Healing shaman were commonly called tube suckers after the type of rituals practiced by them. If a person became sick the healing shaman would visit him alone in the privacy of his lodge. After ascertaining where in the body the ailment was he would take out his paraphernalia consisting of a bowl, three or four hollowed out bones about the size of a child's finger and a rattle. He would begin by chanting to the cadence of his rattle with this ritual gaining all the while in boisterous sounds. This was done to invoke his personal muneedoo who would instruct him as to the exact nature of the ailment and the proper medicines to use. He would then take one of the bones called tubes and place one end on the person's

---

[36] For a complete description of the *Midéwiwin* Lodge and its ceremonies see Johnston, *Ojibway Heritage*, 80-93.

body where the sickness was believed to reside. The shaman would then suck on the tube and spit the infection in the bowl. He would repeat this ritual until the bile contained little or no blood. Meanwhile, outside of the lodge other members of the village would support the shaman by drumming and chanting for their own muneedoog to aid in the healing.

The following records the healing of a Wisconsin Ahnishenahbi youth by a traditional shaman named Old Man Hay using the tube sucking ritual. The testimony is youth's whose name was Tom Badger. He was suffering severe pains in his side.

> In the evening Old Man Hay started to doctor me. He used those bones to doctor me. First he told me to lay on my left side. Then he put the bone right on the place where my pain was. He put his head down close and kept pushing as hard as he could on that bone. When he put the bone away finally, the skin pulled back. That's when it hurt most of all. He started twice to doctor me. The second time he did the same thing he did the first time. When a sucking doctor starts to cure, he first tells the people there about the dream he had at the time he was fasting. Old Man Hay did that. Then my father beat a War Dance drum. Old Man Hay shook a rattle while he doctored me. He put a little dish next to him, with a little water in it. The two bones were lying there. They were about one and a half to two inches long. He didn't touch them with his hands but picked them up with his mouth. He didn't even have to pick them up with his mouth. His power was so strong that when Old Man Hay leaned over the dish, the bones stood up and moved towards his mouth. He swallowed the bones

twice and coughed them up again. Then he put the bone to my side. After he'd finished sucking, Old Man Hay drew out some stuff and spat it into a dish; it looked like blood. Old Man Hay showed it to me and to the others and then threw it into the fire. If he hadn't drawn the blood out it would have turned to pus. And sometimes, when the pus burst inside, the person dies. My father drummed all the time that Old Man Hay was doctoring me. He didn't sing, but Old Man Hay sang a little bit at the beginning of every time he doctored me. He put the bone to my side four times and got blood each time, but the last time he doctored me there was very little blood. It was the same every time he doctored me. All we gave him was a piece of cloth and some tobacco, and gave him his meals. After he had finished doctoring me, Old Man Hay said to my father, "One time they had a medicine dance. You took the hide that Tom got in the medicine dance and gave it to someone else. You promised to give him another one in place of the one you took from him. Sometimes he thinks about it. That's why he is sick now."[37]

The nanandawi was not the only one to practice healing, although he would be called for more serious conditions. The common people also had a fairly comprehensive knowledge of the healing properties of herbs and plants (see appendix 4). These could be used by anyone to cure common ailments and were still used by my family when I was growing up. I have many fond memories of cruising the side roads in the family

[37] John A. Grim, *The Shaman* (Norman, OK: University of Oklahoma Press, 1983), 107-108.

Model-A Ford collecting pennyroyal from the sides of ditches and hanging it in wreathes to dry in the basement. This provided medicine until the following season.

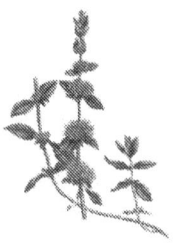

Figure 4—Pennyroyal

A young boy's father who was desperate once visited my father. His son had an ulcerated sore on his foot that would not heal. The leading doctor in the county wanted to amputate. This boy's love was music and he played an instrument in a marching band. The thought of losing that was more than he could bear. They asked my father if he knew of any traditional medicine that might possibly help. For them it was a last resort.

My father prepared a poultice made of a mixture of clay and loam mixed with water and slippery elm bark. He heated it and applied it to the running sore changing it regularly. The sore began to heal and after a few days his doctor pronounced him healed. This story was common knowledge in our family and often told when I was young. Years later I was humbled when I met this very man. He related the same story from his point of view thanking me profusely for my father "saving his foot".

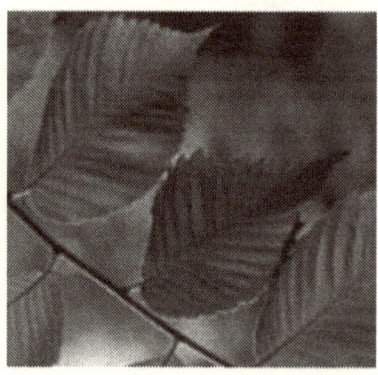

Figure 5—Slippery Elm

The divining shaman, called jiiskiiwnini, communed with the muneedoog while in a trance state. He did this while in a small lodge, called a jiiskaan, specifically constructed for this purpose. This lodge is commonly called a shaking tent and the jiiskiiwnini a shaker. He would perform this ceremony in order to divine some information that remained hidden. For example, an individual or a community might call for a shaker to help find something or someone who was lost. The shaker would perform the shaking tent ceremony to elicit information on the location of the lost item or person. The ceremony was performed in the following manner.

The shaker would prepare for the ceremony either by purifying himself in a sweat lodge, make an offering to his personal muneedoo or smoke some sacred tobacco. The purpose of this preliminary rite was to induce a dream validation in which he would be given the proper symbols to chant and their meaning. These were inscribed on a piece of birch bark and kept. Only he understood the meaning of the symbols and the proper words to chant for each one. This invocation chant would be performed in order to prepare the shaker for the shaking tent ceremony. First his own spirit patron would be invoked and he would undergo an inner transformation that allowed him to be an intermediary figure himself. He then would consciously relate this transformation to the Midéwiwin Lodge so as not to personalize it, which would distort the spiritual power that had entered him. He would now be ready to bring together this power with his traditional mystical knowledge in the shaking tent ceremony he was about to perform.

Meanwhile his assistants would construct a shaking tent by inserting four poles into the ground supported by four crosspieces tied about 2 feet intervals up the vertical poles. One of the vertical posts is higher then the other three by a couple of feet and had the branches left on the top. The wood used to construct the lodge was usually pine. The pine needles at the top of the higher post acted as a conduit for the muneedoog to enter the shaking tent. The top of the lodge was left open but the sides were covered with bark except for a small door through which the shaker entered the tent. A string of bells were sometimes tied between two of the posts.

After dusk when the spiritual readiness of both the shaker and the spiritual world converged the shaker entered the tent and began to drum. There may be drumming also done by the villagers. This was done to induce a trance state in the shaker and to summon the muneedoog into the tent. When they arrived the tent would begin to shake and all drumming would cease. Multiple voices and sparks of light coming from within the tent would also confirm their presence. The shaker would respond to questions from the villagers outside the tent by interpreting the muneedoog' words, which would be spoken in archaic Ahnishenahbewissin. The shaker using this ceremony would ascertain the location of the lost item or person.

Death Customs

There were two ceremonies performed by the Midéwiwin shaman, the funeral rite and the Feast of the Dead. Sometimes, if the person was at the brink of death, the funeral rite was begun before the sick or injured person died. If this were the case the family would take care to dress the person in his or her finest clothing. The weakened person's hair would be impeccably fixed and adorned with feathers. Personal belongings would be laid out beside the body. These would include all the items that person would have used in daily life. A warrior would have placed by his side his war club, knife, musket, ball and shot, flint and tinder, his finest blanket, his pipe and tobacco, a bowl and spoon and his medicine pouch. A woman would have placed at her side her medicine bag, blanket, comb, flint and tinder, cooking utensils, bowl and spoon and sewing gear. These items would be needed for the long journey on the Path of Souls. This led to the Land of Souls where he or she would be reunited with loved ones and friends that had gone on before this death. This place was believed to be located somewhere in the west and was a place of peace and plenty. As the person lie dying the shaman would chant with the cadence of his rattle continuously keeping any evil muneedoo away. The women attending would wail and mourn loudly when the person was unconscious, but if that person regained consciousness they would stop. The men did not mourn out loud.

A warrior would be placed in the sitting position at or just after death, as this was the position he would be buried in. The shaman would speak to the soul of the dead person by chanting instructions while the soul undergoes a change in essence to spirit. He would then leave for a time but the mourners would stay with the body lamenting all the time except for a few of the men who would go off to dig the grave, which would only be four or five feet deep.

When the grave was readied the men would return to join the lamentations. Eventually the shaman would return and chant instructions to the spirit to prepare him for his four-day journey to the Land of Souls. These instructions would include warnings of the dangers to expect on the journey. He would then relate to the people the stories of the origins of the ceremonies, stories of the Path of Souls and stories of the Land of Souls. When he was finished the internment would begin the next morning. The family of the deceased would gather all manner of gifts such as grain, pelts, and other trade goods and place them near the grave.

The Ahnishenahbek used four pallbearers who would carry the bark-encased body to the gravesite. The shaman, the women attendants and all the mourners would accompany them. A fire would be lit and kept going for four days. The body would be placed in the grave facing west with his or her possessions at their feet. The shaman would chant a hymn of benediction and the men would fill the grave with earth. A grave post would be planted at the head of the grave with the person's totem etched on it and perhaps some other markings representing extraordinary deeds. A small grave house made of bark would be constructed over the grave about 30 inches high and the length of the grave. It would have a small entrance on the west end of the house for the spirit of the deceased to exit to the Path of Souls. The gifts brought earlier were moved to the front of the grave house and the women would light a small fire. The mourners would all sit in a circle and during this vigil some of the relatives and close friends would stand and give a eulogy when they felt the need to do so. This continued for four days with attendants tending the grave and keeping the fire going. At the end of the fourth day the shaman, attendants, and gravediggers would be paid in trade goods. The deceased's soul having completed its transformation to spirit could now begin the long journey to the Land of Souls.

While this journey took place a period of celebration would commence with one of the men stepping forward with a small stick in his hand. He would toss it to the crowd and all would try to catch it. One would but the others would try to wrestle it away from him. This continued until all or most had handled the stick and when one finally held fast to the stick he would be awarded some prize. It then would be announced that another prize would be awarded to the winner of a footrace. All the young men would line themselves in a single line across the start and race on a predetermined course to the designated finish line.

After these celebratory activities the people would return to the village where the relatives would give a feast for all mourners that were not relatives nor related by marriage. They were informed that the deceased was providing for the feast and a small piece of food from this feast must be taken by the guests and placed at the grave. They then returned to the village where they could eat as much as they wanted and they were also allowed to take the rest of their portions home with them. The guests of the feast are then given considerable presents, thanked and congratulated on their own generosity.

The widow or widower would enter a period of mourning that would last for one year. A widow would move into the lodge of her husband's parents for the mourning period. She would wear her hair down and not braided. She replaced her good dress with an old worn one and she would wear a sash over her left shoulder and tied at her right hip. Her good dress folded and placed in a birch bark pouch, which was tied to her waist. Any gifts she received during the mourning period would be added to this bundle. She was required to attend her husband's grave every a day until released from the mourning period. At the end of the year she would ask her husband's parents to release her from her outward mourning after which she would replace the worn dress with her good one, be able to use the gifts held in her birch bark pouch and would be free to remarry.

The living were responsible for the care of the dead. The graves were tended regularly during a three-year cycle, but at the end of the cycle a Feast of the Dead would be held. At this time a special lodge would be built about 120 feet long, open on the top and with several tiers running along the insides of it. It would be constructed using fresh bark only and have three long poles planted one at each end and a taller one in the centre. They would be painted and greased and have a prize attached to the top each of them. The prize would belong to the first person to be able to scale the pole and touch the prize.

After this contest each family would disinter the bodies of their relatives, clean the bones and place them in birch bark containers bringing them to the lodge and placing them on the ledges. They then heaped all the gifts they had collected during the three years on the remains. With faces painted black they would partake of a great feast, which they would leave occasionally returning to the lodge where they would circle making a great noise by shooting muskets in the air and bellowing loud whoops. They would then return to the feast to eat some more. Back and forth the mourners would go all the while making a din of noise for three days and three nights. At the end of this time the relatives would retrieve the gifts from the lodge and distributed them to the guests that were not relatives.

They then retrieved the bones from the lodge after which the men circled the lodge one more time shouting their mourning whoops and striking the structure with large poles knocking it to pieces. At the same time the women threw bundles of kindling on the collapsed lodge and it was burned. As an anti-climax a Dog Feast was held where a great number of dogs were killed and feasted upon. Dogs were highly regarded by the village and deemed appropriate as a sacrifice to offer up prayers for the dead. After the Dog Feast the relatives took the bones to a desolate place where they were hidden in hollows or between rocks. The dead were never spoken of again. This was the climax to the Feast of the Dead and served as final closure for the living.

Appendices

Appendix 1—Clan Systems

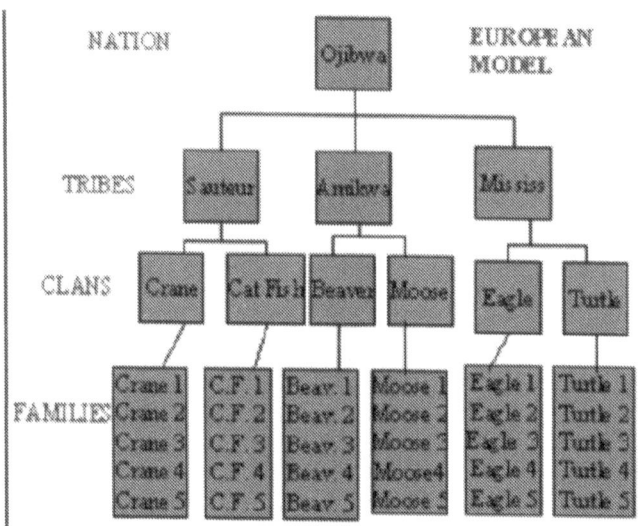

FIRST NATIONS MODEL

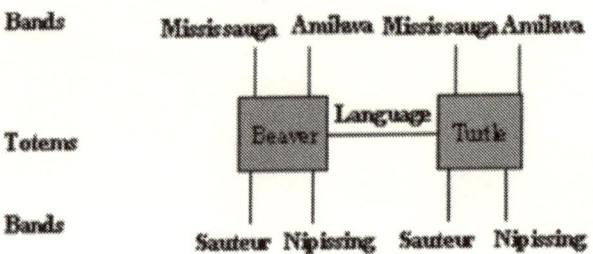

Appendix 2—Chief Yellowhead's Speech[38]

Chief Yellowhead rose up and made a speech and exhibited the great Wampum belt of the Six Nations, and explained the talk contained in it. This Wampum was about 3 feet long and 4 inches wide. It had a row of White Wampum in the centre, running from one end to the other, and the representations of wigwams every now and then, and a large round Wampum tied neatly in the middle of the Belt, with a representation of the sun in the centre. Yellowhead stated that this Belt was given by the Nahdooways (Haudenosaunee) to the Ojebways (Anishnaabeg) many years ago—about the time the French first came to this country. That the great Council took place at Lake Superior—That the Nahdooways made the road or path and pointed out the different council fires which were to be kept lighted. The first marks on the Wampum represented that a council fire should be kept burning at the Sault St. Marie. The 2nd mark represented the Council fire at the Manitoulin Island, where a beautiful White fish was placed, who should watch the fire as long as the world stood. The 3rd mark represented the Council fire placed on and Island opposite Penetanguishene Bay, on which was placed a Beaver to watch the fire. The 4th mark represents the Council fire lighted up at the Narrows of Lake Simcoe at which place was put a White Rein Deer. To him the Rein Deer was committed the keeping of this Wampum talk. At this place our fathers hung up the Sun, and said that the Sun should be a witness to all what had been done and that when any of their descendents saw the Sun they might remember the acts of their forefathers. At the Narrows our fathers placed a

---

[38] NAC, RG10, Volume 1011.

dish with ladles around it, and a ladle from the Six Nations, who said to the Ojebways that the dish or bowl should never be emptied, but he (Yellowhead) was sorry to say that it had already been emptied, not by the Six Nations on the Grand River, but by the Caucanawaugas residing near Montreal. The 5th mark represented the Council fire which was placed at this River Credit where a beautiful White headed Eagle was placed upon a very tall pine tree, in order to watch the Council fires and see if any ill winds blew upon the smoke of the Council fires. A dish was also placed at the Credit. That the right of hunting on the north side of the Lake was secured by the Ojebways, and that the Six Nations were not to hunt here only when they come to smoke the pipe of peace with their Ojebway brethren.

Appendix 3[39]—Midéwiwin Ceremony

Having been informed that the Indians were about to attend a Medai Kechewegoondewin, or Conjurers great feast, I determined if practicable, to witness the ceremony: first, for my own satisfaction; and secondly, with the view of furnishing the readers of the Guardian with the particulars.

This feast was given, and the ceremony attended to, in order to initiate two Indian children into the order of Medai or Conjurors, or as some writers on Indian customs have been pleased to designate this class of men, the "priesthood". The ground selected for this occasion, was a sandy spot on the bank of the St. Clair River, about half a mile distant from the Mission house, close by the graves of the sleeping fathers of this once numerous tribe; a spot for which the Indians generally have a great veneration.

Early in the morning of the day appointed, the women assembled, with implements suitable for their labour, and levelled the ground, carefully removing all the small stumps and roots, and making the same perfectly smooth. Small stakes, at regular distances, were driven into the ground, enclosing a plot of about fifty feet in length and 25 in breadth, to these at the height of about 5 feet were tied with bark, long poles, to which were hung canoe-sails, tent cloths, blankets, etc.; thus enclosing the whole, and excluding observations and entrance, except at each end where an opening of about 6 feet was left. In the

---

[39] Rev. James Evans, Christian Guardian, 28 January 1835 45, reprinted in Elizabeth Graham, Medicine Man to Missionary (Toronto: P. Martin Associates, 1975), appendix 2, 98-104.

centre were driven two strong stakes about two feet apart, to each of which was tied a wooden image resembling the human figure, the head being loose in order to admit the body which was below, to be filled, as it was on this occasion, with kahskeken or medicine prepared from roots, barks, leaves, etc.

About noon, nine kettles, holding from two to four pails full, were placed before the company; some few were served from the same in tin pans but the greater part, unceremoniously, and in no small quantities, helped themselves. And the pork, hams, venison, ducks, squirrels, raccoons, bears meat and other game being boiled to shreds they found no difficulty in dispensing with forks, and in many cases with knives also, pulling the food to pieces, and appearing to comprehend the old proverb, "fingers were made before forks:" nor were they less forgetful of the Indian maxim "eat all that is set before you:" for it can scarcely be said the kettles were successively emptied, – but rather simultaneously; the company amounted to between one hundred and fifty and two hundred.   This evidently gratifying part of the ceremony being ended, a select party consisting of the Medai or Conjurors, retired to the woods and spent nearly an hour in singing to the spirits; while the women fetched some straw and spread it around the enclosure, and made some other necessary arrangements.   As the evening shadows closed in, the fires were lighted, one at each entrance, and the company began to take their seats. After some time, for Indian movements are generally very deliberately performed, all were seated, and one of the Medai took the Tatewaegun or drum and commenced slowly beating it at intervals of nearly a second, as a signal that all was now in readiness; upon which the men, women and children arose, and took their places in rows or rank within the enclosure; this done, the Medai began to beat more lively, two women accompanying the sound of the drum with the sheshegwun or rattle, while they struck a song and all began to dance; this consisted in a gentle and not ungraceful movement of the body, and occasionally a step or two with the feet. So regular and uniform is the movement and so grotesque the appearance, each being wrapped in a new white blanket, on which being a beautiful clear night, the moon, which was full, cast her silver light and gave a striking effect to the scene, that an observer can scarcely believe but that the ground on which he stands is in motion, and almost imagine himself to be moving in unison with the company. There were present nine male and two female Medin, the drum was alternately beat and the singing led by each about half an hour, while all joined in the chorus; the men occasionally singing softly, unaccompanied by the females, and at other times having pleasant voices, they produce, unassociated with the recollection of paganism, not unpleasing music. This was the introduction to the ceremony of initiation. A little boy about six and a little girl about seven years of age were the subjects; these, who had accompanied the Medai to the words, now joined in the singing, and took a prominent place in the dance. After this dance, the drum having been beat by each Medai, all took their seats, and each took a dram of whiskey...

A blanket was now spread in the centre, and the two children were seated thereon, with their faces towards the images before mentioned; and pieces of blue and red cloth, containing about a quarter of a yard each were spread at their feet. Two women took their places behind them, in the parts they would be required to act in the ceremony. The oldest man in the tribe arose and spoke about fifteen minutes, addressing himself first to the men, then to the women and lastly to the children. Exhorting them to hold facts on the religion of their fathers; to be patient in enduring hardships; and urging on the children to observe mahgahtawin or blacking and fasting; (a religious ceremony) and closed by promising them, should they observe what he said, beards as white as his, which was silvered over with age and limbs as strong therewith; he then began a song in praise of the children seated in the centre, the chorus, in which all joined being: "Oh, Oh nejahnesun, ne nejahnesun" which ended all at once arose, crying "Wah wah wah" and commenced dancing and moving around the enclosure in file, keeping in their movements the most regular order, and timing their steps to the drums, rattles and vocal sounds. This exercise, which appeared to be a compliment to the children, all the song being in their praise, continued about fifteen or twenty minutes, and again all resumed their seats.

The Medai now arose, all the rest remaining seated in silence, and each took his or her kahshkekeh mahahkemoot, or medicine pouch, being an otter skin, containing from fifty to a hundred very small parcels of mahshkekeh, or medicine used in conjuring, consisting of roots, leaves, bark, cinnamon cloves, tobacco, a small wooden box, some mekis, or sea shells, a wooden snake, some porcupine quills, a mink or squirrel skin, also full of medicine, atahpejegun, or cord to tie prisoners in war, a sheshegwun, or rattle used in curing the sick; and a variety of other small articles – and hung it in the belt around the waist. The chief Medai taking the lead, the others following, walked slowly and majestically around the enclosure several times, the chief Medai pressing on them to attend to their duty on this occasion; after which each took his pouch from the belt in which it hung, and singing, kept the head of the skin moving up and down, thus beating time to their song. In a few minutes, continuing singing, they moved in file dancing towards the two children, carrying their skins in both hands, and giving them a gently undulating movement, similar to that of a snake in motion; each as he arrived presented the head of the skin to one and then to the other of the children's breasts, crying, "Hahwah yahwah." And at each presentation the women threw the children on their faces, raising them again for the next until the last, when the children were both left on their faces as if dead. All now uttered as loudly as possible, "Wah wah wah and quickly retreated in haste, as if afraid, to the end of the enclosure; the women, at the same time stooping down and applying their mouths to the ears of the children, called aloud, "Ahwah ahwah ahwah" repeating these sounds five times; and pointing north, east, south and west, and lastly into the ground, again cried, "Wah wah wah" and raised the children to a sitting posture. The Medai during this time continued singing and walking slowly around the enclosure until they arrived again opposite the children, where they all stood still with their mouths open, and the chief Medai took from his pouch a root, and breaking it into small pieces put into each Medai's mouth a piece, which was chewed as they danced around. On arriving at the children they successively spat a little of the juice on the breast, on each side the neck, and on the back of each of the children; walking around once more, they each took up the pieces of cloth which laid by the children, and muttered some words too low to be distinguished, and retired to the end of the ground. Here they commenced singing and taking their skins, gave them the undulating motion before mentioned; then they proceeded to the children from whom they retreated in haste, and fell one over the other at the entrance of the enclosure. In a little time they arose, placed themselves in a row, and looking directly upwards, their heads being thrown back as far as possible, each holding in his finger and thumb a small piece of mahskekeh, he put it five times into his own mouth, at each time crying "Yahahwah, Yahahwah, Yahahwah" and pointing to the four points and into the ground as before mentioned, they ran and fell at the other end of the encampment.

Each Medai now arose and made a speech, declaring the children to be regularly received into their community and to be constituted Medai, and that they should in future have the privilege of joining in every Medaiwegoontewin, and enjoining on each other to embrace every opportunity of instructing them in the wisdom of the Medai and promising them if these children endeavour to become wise, and attend to mahkahtiwin, (blacking and fasting) they would always own them as brethren among the Medai.   The children were now led around the ground by their attendant women, and their right hands presented to every one present, the women shewing to everyone a small sea shell; after which all joined in singing and dancing...

J. EVANS, St. Clair Rapids   18th Dec. 1834.

Appendix 4—Medicines[40]

Aamjiwnaang Territory[41] Traditional Medicines

English Name
American Elder

Latin Name
Sambucus Canadensis

Description
Branching shrub found throughout Aamjiwnaang Territory.

Medicinal Use
Make a tea from shrub's flowers for babies suffering from colic.

---

[40] Regarding traditional medicines the information presented herein is for informational purposes only. The results reported may not necessarily occur in all individuals. For many of the conditions discussed, treatment with prescription or over-the-counter medication is also available. Consult your doctor, practitioner, and/or pharmacist for any health problem and before using any traditional remedies or before making any changes in prescribed medications.

[41] Aamjiwnaang Territory included all of St. Clair, Lapeer, Genesee and Shiawasseeand parts of Sanilac, Tuscola and Saginaw counties in Michigan, all of Perth and parts of Lambton, Huron, Middlesex, Waterloo, Oxford, Wellington counties in Ontario.

English Name
Beech

Latin Name
Fagus Grandifolia

Description
This large tree with smooth bark can be found throughout Aamjiwnaang Territory.

Medicinal Use
Same as American Elder.

English Name
Black-eyed Susan

Latin Name
Rudbeckia Hirta

Description
Common wild flower found throughout Aamjiwnaang Territory.

Medicinal Use
Make a root tea and drink for colds.

English Name
Boneset

Latin Name
Eupatorium Perfoliatum

Description
Hairy stemmed weed one to three feet high with white flowers. Found throughout Aamjiwnaang Territory.

Medicinal Use
Collect leaves and flowering tops while in bloom, make tea

for fever, body pains and colds.

English Name   **Latin Name**
  Butterfly Milkweed   Asclepias Tuberosa

Description
  Erect stem one to two feet high, thick growth of leaves and bright orange flowers followed by edible seeds. Widespread in Aamjiwnaang Territory but not in Huron, Perth or Oxford counties.

Medicinal Use
  Chew fresh root for bronchitis or other respiratory complaints.

English Name   **Latin Name**
  Butternut   Juglans Cinerea

Description
  Large tree belonging to the walnut family found throughout Aamjiwnaang Territory.

Medicinal Use
  The syrup can be eaten for digestive disorders or make a tea of the bark and drink for upset stomach or as a laxative.

English Name   **Latin Name**
  Canada Anemone   Anemone Canadensis

Description

Found throughout Aamjiwnaang Territory.

Medicinal Use

Same as Butternut.

English Name	**Latin Name**
Canada Fleabane	Erigeron Canadensis

Description

A common weed can grow to ten feet, has hairy leaves and small white flowers found throughout Aamjiwnaang Territory.

Medicinal Use

Burn this weed in a smudge pot inside the lodge to produce a smoke that is an excellent insect repellent.

English Name	**Latin Name**
Canada Goldenrod	Solidago Candensis

Description

Common wild flower found Aamjiwnaang Territory.

Medicinal Use

Chew blossoms and slowly swallow juices to relieve sore throat.

English Name	**Latin Name**

Eastern Hemlock   Tsuga Canadensis

Description

Large coniferous tree found throughout Aamjiwnaang Territory.

Medicinal Use

Prepare tea from inner bark and drink to relieve cold symptoms and influenza.

English Name   Latin Name

Highbush Cranberry   Virburnum Opulus

Description

A small tree up to ten feet in height with broad oval leaves, white flowers and sour red fruit.   Found throughout Aamjiwnaang Territory.

Medicinal Use

Treat mumps by drinking an infusion of the bark.

English Name   Latin Name

Lady's Slipper   Cypripendium

Description

Member of the orchid family with erect stem one to two feet high, large oval leaves and a single yellow flower found throughout Aamjiwnaang Territory.

Medicinal Use

Dig rhizome and roots in fall, clean with water and dry in the shade. Make a powder of the dried root and use one teaspoon per cup of water. Drink for insomnia.

English Name	**Latin Name**
Mullein	Verbascum Thapsus

Description

Common pasture weed introduced from Europe grows up to seven feet with thick rough velvety leaves and yellow flowers. Found throughout Aamjiwnaang Territory.

Medicinal Use

Leaves are smoked for relief from Asthma.

English Name	**Latin Name**
Multi-coloured Blue-flag Iris	Iris Versicolor

Description

Common Iris had violet flowers with yellow green and white stripes and is found throughout Aamjiwnaang Territory.

Medicinal Use

Boil root and pound to pulp. Apply to bruised and swollen area then rinse later with water used in boiling.

English Name

Panicled Dogwood

Latin Name

Cornus Paniculata

Description

Shrub or small tree found throughout Aamjiwnaang Territory.

Medicinal Use

Pound the inner bark and insert the compressed mass into the anus to cure hemorrhoids.

English Name

Pennyroyal

Latin Name

Hedeoma Pulegioides

Description

Aromatic plant not more than one foot in height with small opposite leaves on short stems and pale blue flowers found throughout Aamjiwnaang Territory.

Medicinal Use

Steep leaves and drink tea for upset stomach, headache or to induce sweating at the first sign of a cold.

English Name

Pine

Latin Name

Pinus

Description

Coniferous tree found mainly in Lambton, Sanilac and St. Clair counties but also found sparsely throughout Aamjiwnaang

Territory.

Medicinal Use

Salve made of pine gum, wax and animal fat. Apply to boils, sores, cuts and wounds.

English Name	Latin Name
Prairie Buttercup	Ranunculus Rhomboideus

Description

Root puts forth several slender stems which flower at its ends. Restricted to Lambton Middlesex and St. Clair counties of Aamjiwnaang Territory..

Medicinal Use

Plant is poisonous and should be used externally only. Pulverize the root, soak in warm water and apply wash over wounds and cuts.

English Name	Latin Name
Purple Boneset	Eupatorium Purpureum

Description

From three to ten feet tall with leaves in whorls of three to six and numerous white to pink or purple flowers. Found throughout Aamjiwnaang Territory.

Medicinal Use

Used as an aphrodisiac and nibbled on when opposite sex

converse.

English Name
Sassafras

Latin Name
Sassafras Albidum

Description
Large aromatic tree found in the Carolinian forests of Aamjiwnaang Territory.

Medicinal Use
Steep roots to make an infusion. Drink liquid to treat measles and associated fever.

English Name
Seneca Snakeroot

Latin Name
Polygala Senega

Description
Each root puts up as many as twenty slender stems up to one foot high and has small greenish white flowers. Widespread in Aamjiwnaang Territory but not found in Huron, Perth or Oxford counties.

Medicinal Use
Collect roots in fall. Chew roots and apply directly to snake bites or boil whole plant and drink for diarrhea or respiratory ailments. **DO NOT OVERDOSE** as plant is poisonous.

English Name

Latin Name

Slippery Elm   Ulmus Fulva

Description

Large tree with broad flat topped crown and large rough leaves and dark brown, deep furrowed bark found throughout Aamjiwnaang Territory.

Medicinal Use

Make a tea from the inner bark and drink for sore throat. Inner bark can also be mixed with common earth to make a poultice and apply to open sores or wounds.

English Name   **Latin Name**

Smooth Sumac   Rhus Glabra

Description

Grows from large shrub to small tree with small fruit in large red clusters found throughout Aamjiwnaang Territory.

Medicinal Use

Boil leaves and pour decoction over frostbitten area. Also a fresh root can be chewed to cure mouth sores.

English Name   **Latin Name**

Spikenard   Aralia Racemosa

Description

Grows to six feet with large alternate leaves with small greenish flowers and small reddish purple fruit. Found throughout Aamjiwnaang Territory.

Medicinal Use

Make a tea of the roots and drink for backache.

English Name	Latin Name
Spotted Jewel-weed	Impatiens Capensis

Description

Five to six feet high with yellow flowers, capsules burst and curl at touch. Found throughout Aamjiwnaang Territory.

Medicinal Use

Apply juice from leaves to relieve itch from poison ivy or oak. Crush leaves and stems and apply to rash or eczema.

English Name	Latin Name
Stiff Goldenrod	Solidago Rigida

Description

Restricted wild flower found only in Lambton, Middlesex, Perth and St. Clair counties of Aamjiwnaang Territory.

Medicinal Use

Grind the flowers into a lotion and apply to insect bites and stings.

English Name

Sunflower

Latin Name

Helianthus Annuus

Description

Common wild flower found throughout Aamjiwnaang Territory.

Medicinal Use

Crush the root and apply mash in a wet dressing to draw blisters.

English Name

Thimbleweed

Latin Name

Anemone Cylindrica

Description

Erect perennial herb widespread but not in Huron, Perth or Oxford counties.

Medicinal Use

Boil the root then pound to make a wash. Apply directly to wounds or make a tea from roots and drink for headache.

English Name

White Oak

Latin Name

Quercus Alba

Description

Large deciduous tree found throughout Aamjiwnaang Territory.

Medicinal Use

Boil the bark and drink the liquid for bleeding piles and diarrhea. Inner bark is a powerful antiseptic.

English Name	Latin Name
Wild Bergamot	Monarda Fistulosa

Description

Slender stem two to three feet high with lilac to pink flowers and thin oval leaves. Found throughout Aamjiwnaang Territory.

Medicinal Use

Boil dried plant to extract oil and breath in for bronchitis and colds. Oil collected can also be used to dry up pimples.

English Name	Latin Name
Wild Black Cherry	Prunus Serotina

Description

A large tree with white flowers found throughout Aamjiwnaang Territory.

Medicinal Use

Collect root bark in the fall and steep to make a tea and use as a sedative.

English Name	Latin Name
Wild Carrot	Daucus Carota

Description

Also known as Queen Anne's Lace it grows from one to three feet with large white flowers. It is found throughout Aamjiwnaang Territory.

Medicinal Use

Steep blossoms in warm water and drink for diabetes.

English Name	Latin Name
Wild Mint	Mentha Arvensis

Description

Has whorled flowers borne in axils of leaves and smells like peppermint. Found throughout Aamjiwnaang Territory.

Medicinal Use

Make a decoction from dried leaves and stems. Drink the liquid for nausea and vomiting.

English Name	Latin Name
Wild Plum	Prunus Americana

Description

A thicket-forming shrub or small tree with white flowers and red plums found in Lambton and St. Clair counties of Aamjiwnaang Territory.

Medicinal Use

Boil the scrapped inner bark and gargle the solution to cure mouth sores or drink a tea made from the roots to expel intestinal worms.

English Name   **Latin Name**
  Willow   Salix

Description
  Pussy willow is found throughout Aamjiwnaang Territory.

Medicinal Use
  Apply a solution made from the leaves and young twigs to itchy scalp and to remove dandruff. Also boil the bark and drink to reduce fever and relieve pain.

English Name   **Latin Name**
  Witch Hazel   Hamamelis Virginiana

Description
  Slightly aromatic shrub or small tree with small yellow flowers found throughout Aamjiwnaang Territory.

Medicinal Use
  Boil the leaves and rub liquid on aching muscles or use twigs in the water of a sweat lodge to make steam for muscular aches.

English Name   **Latin Name**
  Yarrow   Achillea Millefolium

Description

Common weed found throughout Aamjiwnaang Territory.

Medicinal Use

Steep whole plant and pour liquid in ear for earache or crush between stones and apply to minor wounds.

English Name	**Latin Name**
Yellow Nut-Grass	Cyperus Esculentus

Description

Perennial grass found throughout Aamjiwnaang Territory.

Medicinal Use

Pound the tubers of the grass with tobacco leaves. Apply in a wet dressing for athlete's foot.

Abbreviations

AGA	Art Gallery of Algoma
MHS	Minnesota Historical Society
MPHSC	Michigan Pioneer Historical Collections
NAC	National Archives of Canada
NARA	United States National Archives and Research Administration
NYCD	New York Colonial Documents
OVGLEA:MC	Ohio Valley-Great Lakes Ethnohistory Archives: Miami Collection

ROM	Royal Ontario Museum
SAAM	Smithsonian American Art Museum
WHS	Wisconsin Historical Society

Illustration Credits

SAAM. Ball players by George Catlin, year unknown. Hand coloured lithograph on paper. Photo image courtesy of Wikimedia Commons.

ROM. Ojibwa camp on Lake Huron, on the shores of Georgian Bay. Field sketch by Paul Kane (1810—1871), 1845. Pencil on paper, 13.7×21.7 cm. Photo image courtesy of Wikimedia Commons.

Ojibwa wigwam. Detail from a painting (1846) by Paul Kane of an Ojibwa village at Sault Ste. Marie. Photo image courtesy of Wikimedia Commons.

WHS. "Chippewas Gathering Wild Rice". Illustration of three Chippewas gathering wild rice in a canoe. Artist unknown. Negative No. WHi 5599.

ROM. "Spearing Salmon by Torchlight". An oil painting by Paul Kane Photo Image courtesy of Wikimedia Commons.

WHS. "Indian Sugar Camp" Drawn by Captain Seth Eastman, U.S. Army ca. 1850. Negative No. Negative No. WHi 9829.

"The Snowshoe Dance" by George Catlin 1835. Photo image courtesy of Wikimedia Commons.

"Dance to the Berdache" by George Catlin. Photo image courtesy Wikimedia Commons.

AGA. Hole in the Sky, 1981, Andrew Dutkewych. Photo image courtesy of Wikimedia Commons.

Pipe Tomahawk photo by D. F. Barry between 1854-1930. Photo image courtesy of Wikimedia Commons.

MHS. "Building Birch Bark Canoe at a Chippewa Camp" by Truman Ward Ingersol ca. 1895. Loc. No. E97.35 Negative No. 2178.
.

WHS. Shaking Tent in the WHS Visual Archives: Negative No. WHi (x3) 6031.

Father Jacques Marque (Jesuit Missionary 1637-1675). Photo image courtesy Wikimedia Commons.

NARA. One-Called-From-A-Distance (Midéwiwin), an Ahnishenahbi medicine-man from White Earth Reservation, Minnesota, 1894. Photo image courtesy of Wikimedia Commons.

SELECTED BIBLIOGRAPHY

Benton-Banai, Edward. The Mishomis Book. Hayward, WI: Indian Country Communication, Inc., 1988.

Blackbird, Andrew J. History of the Ottawa and Chippewa Indians of Michigan. Ypsilanti, MI: The Ypsilanti Job Printing House, 1887 available at http://www.canadiana.org/ECO/PageView?id=a31b3e758 e50350b&display=00429+0003 last accessed 27 June 2006.

Champlain, Samuel de, Voyages of Samuel de Champlain 1537-1635, Vol. 1, trans. Charles Pomeroy Otis Ph.D. Boston: The Prince Society, 1880, available from http://www.canadiana.org/ECO/ItemRecord/26911?id=6 08edce981ea4d7a last accessed 20 July 2006.

Copway, G. The Traditional History and Characteristics of the Ojibway Nation. London: Charles Gilpin, 1850 available from http://www.canadiana.org/eco/english/index.html

last accessed 18 July 2006.

Gold , Reuben Thwaites ed   The Jesuit Relations and Allied
    Documents, 71 vols. Clevland: The Burrows Brothers
    Publishing, Latter nineteenth century.

Grim, John A. The Shaman. Norman, OK: University of
    Oklahoma Press, 1983.

Johnston, Basil. The Manitous.Toronto: Key Porter Books Ltd.,
    1995

Johnston, Basil. Ojibway Ceremonies.Toronto: McClellan and
    Stewart, 1982. Reprinted 1987.

Johnston, Basil. Ojibway Heritage. Toronto: McClellan and
    Stewart, 1976, Reprinted 1994.

Jones, Rev. Peter. History of the Ojebway Indians; With
    Especial Reference to Their Conversion to Christianity.
    London: A.W. Bennett, 1861 available from
    http://www.canadiana.org/ECO/ItemRecord/35737?id=b
    0fa8e3c6abfb66d last accessed 6 July 2006.

Kinietz, Vernon W. The Indians of the Western Great Lakes
    1615-1760. Ann Arbor: University of Michigan Press, 1940;
    Ann Arbor Paperbacks, Ann Arbor: 1991.

Kohl, J.G., Kitchi-Gami, Wanderings Around Lake Superior.
    London: Chapman and Hall, 1860 available from
    http://www.canadiana.org/eco/english/index.html   last
    accessed 21 July 2006.

Long, J. Voyages and Travels of an Indian Interpreter and
    Trader. London: J. Long, 1791, facsimile edition, Toronto:
    Coles Publishing Co., 1974.

Mahon, John K. The War of 1812. New York: Da Cappo Press,
    1991.

Plain, Aylmer N. History of the Sarnia Indian Reserve. (Brights
    Grove, ON: G. Smith, 1975), 16 quoted in Schmalz,
    Ojibwa, 212.

Plain, Nicholas. The History of Chippewas of Sarnia and the History of Sarnia Reserve. Sarnia, ON: Privately Printed, 1951.

Rogers Edward S. and Donald B. Smith, ed., Aboriginal Ontario. Toronto: Dundurn Press, 1994.

Strickland, Major C.M., Twenty-seven Years in Canada West or The Experience of an Early Settler, ed. Agnes Strickland, 2 Vols. London: Richard Bentley Publisher, 1853 available from   http://www.canadiana.org/eco/english/index.html last accessed 20 July 2006.

Warren, William W. History of the Ojibway People. St. Paul: Minnesota Historical Society Press, vol. 5, 1885; Borealis Books, 1984.